"JUST REMEMBER, DARLING, I'LL SEE TO IT THAT ANYTHING BAD THAT HAPPENS TO ME WILL ALSO HAPPEN TO YOU," NICOLE WARNED . . .

Before she could continue, there was a knock at the door. "Donnie darling, are you expecting someone?" she asked.

"I don't know what to expect anymore," Donnie said sourly. "You're naked," he reminded her. "My robe's hanging in the bathroom." As Nicole went into the bath, he moved to the door and opened it.

"Hello, love of my life!" Sonny, bright-eyed and apple-cheeked, threw her arms around him, backing him into the room. "Ooh, I like a man without a shirt! He's got less to take off before bed! I would have got here earlier—"

She stopped dead. Her eyes widened, and she went pale as she saw Nicole, barely concealed beneath a bath towel, step out of Donnie's bathroom.

"Who is it, darling?" Nicole called out. "Oh! My . . ." Donnie watched helplessly as Nicole, pretending surprise and embarrassment, smiled mockingly at Sonny. "How are you, dear child?"

Books in the HAROLD ROBBINS PRESENTS™ Series

Published by POCKET BOOKS

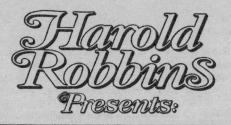

Harold Robbins Presents:

High Performance

A novel by
Lawrence Field

PUBLISHED BY POCKET BOOKS NEW YORK

Another *Original* publication of POCKET BOOKS

POCKET BOOKS, a division of Simon & Schuster, Inc.
1230 Avenue of the Americas, New York, N.Y. 10020

ISBN: 0-671-64083-6

First Pocket Books printing January 1988

10 9 8 7 6 5 4 3 2 1

POCKET and colophon are trademarks of
Simon & Schuster, Inc.

HAROLD ROBBINS PRESENTS is a trademark
of Harold Robbins.

Printed in the U.S.A.

High Performance

1

MORGAN WAS CHATTING with the groom when the bride, immaculate in beaded ivory lace and creamy antique tulle, propositioned him.

Damn, he hated these affairs. Well, actually, he enjoyed affairs. It was parties he hated.

A wedding reception, even one held in honor of the celebrity-infested extravaganza that was Grace Tyler and Matt Palmer's marriage, was just an alias for a party, and Morgan was not a party animal. He'd left San Francisco late last night, pulling into Carmel, where he'd booked a room, a little before dawn. He'd slept a few hours, then showered, and put on a gray Armani suit, a pale blue silk shirt and a black knit tie. The drive from Carmel to the ocean front, Big Sur hideaway of the Hollywood producer who was hosting this reception, took about an hour. Morgan had timed it well, handing over the BMW's keys to the parking valet twenty minutes before the ceremony was scheduled to begin on this balmy, August afternoon.

Now bride and groom—who had already been united in a multimillion dollar movie deal—were united in holy matrimony. A hundred or so guests were crowded onto the landscaped terraces cut like steps into the steep cliffs overlooking the ocean. The crash of the waves against the rocks, combined with the droning clatter of the swooping media helicopters, was making it hard to hear. Morgan was trying to talk with Matt

Palmer about current box office grosses, a subject Morgan knew next to nothing about.

Matt Palmer was wearing a double-breasted, midnight blue tux, a white silk T-shirt, no socks, and black aerobic workout shoes. He was short and slight, with a honey-colored, mile high pompadour. Palmer was upset about the eavesdropping choppers. Morgan didn't blame him. The long, black telescopic lenses pointing down at them looked eerily like gun barrels. But such was the price Palmer had to pay for fame and fortune. On film Palmer projected the volatility and white heat of Cagney in his prime, qualities that had earned him his reputation as Hollywood's hottest bratpacker.

Palmer was still verbally abusing the media when Grace Tyler, regal in her gown and veil, had come up beside Morgan and put her arm around his waist. "This fucking sea breeze is curling the hell out of my haircut," she'd said.

Grace was the platinum blonde star of a box office smash adventure flick about a twenty-first century female police detective. Her new album was at the top of the charts. Morgan had met her back in the seventies, when he was still driving the Grand Prix circuit, and Grace Tyler was still Lucy Mahaney, barely into her late teens, but already a high priced call girl when she wasn't being a "pit popsie"; trading her favors for rides in the low-slung racing machines that set her own libido racing.

Grace's exotic beauty was extraordinary, and particularly impressive to Morgan, who had first hand knowledge of how she had done her best to squander it through the years. She'd lived fast and hard, and yet her beauty was unmarred—unlike Ilsa.

Morgan flashed on the scalding image of how Ilsa had looked at the end, but quickly shook off the bad memories, and his bitterness. Some people are casualties, some people survive, and some people do a lot better than that, he reminded himself. More power to Grace if somewhere along the way she'd learned to airbrush life.

"Wanna kiss the bride?" Grace asked. Morgan obliged her. She tasted of champagne, bubble gum and cocaine.

"Want another?" Grace asked. "I tried to seduce this guy a million times," she confided to her new husband. "All the other guys at the track came on to me, but not Don Morgan."

"I liked it fine that we were friends," Morgan said lightly, trying to turn it all into a joke. Matt Palmer looked uncomfortable. Morgan, watching Grace's darting, glittery eyes, realized drugs and alcohol were doing the talking. He guessed Matt Palmer realized it too, but wondered why the groom didn't take his bride in hand.

"I think it was because you were married," Grace said, nodding. "I know you think I'm pretty." She shrugged. "I mean, *everybody* does, and you certainly *seem* healthy—"

Her hands had slid underneath his jacket. Morgan gently, but firmly removed them from his person. Grace didn't seem to notice. Palmer had suddenly become very pale.

"Yeah, I think it was because Morgan was married," Grace said. "Morgan didn't cheat when he was driving, and he didn't cheat on his wife. I bet he doesn't even cheat in business."

Morgan winked at Palmer. "I guess she means I don't cheat."

"The thing of it is," Grace continued, running her fingers along the line of Morgan's jaw. "You're not married, now."

"Honey," Morgan gently chided, not sure just how wrecked out of her skull she was, "the thing of it is, you *are*."

"Just *barely*, Morgan. It's not too late . . ."

"Jesus Christ, what are you doing?" Palmer at long

3

last exploded. " 'It's not too late.' What the fuck is that supposed to mean?"

"It means, it's not like I'm a virgin!" Grace snapped, advancing angrily on her husband. "What's the big deal?"

"Come'mere, I want to talk to you—" Palmer grabbed her by the wrist and dragged her away.

Morgan glanced at his watch. As soon as his business was done he could get the hell out of here.

"One of the truly great romances of our time," remarked a knockout, curly haired redhead with a thick, French accent. She was wearing a grayish, glen plaid suit trimmed in black velvet. Her skirt was short enough to reveal her lovely legs. She looked beautiful, and familiar; Morgan struggled to place her.

"Tell me, do all brides throw themselves at your feet?"

"I guess I'm just too handsome for my own good," Morgan said.

"It could be a problem for you," she agreed, and walked away.

Morgan watched her go. He still couldn't remember her name, if he'd ever known it, but he couldn't shake the feeling that he'd seen her before. Well, most of the people at the wedding were in show business. Maybe she was as an actress. Maybe he'd seen her in some film.

Morgan checked his Rolex again, wishing the flatbed would get here and unload, so that he could be on his way. The rig had checked in with him on the car phone as he was leaving Carmel; it should have been here by now.

It was time to find a telephone. Morgan had noticed one by the pool, and headed that way, but when he got there it was being used by some guy in one of those unconstructed jacket and baggy pants deals, with his shirt buttoned all the way up to the neck and no tie. Morgan waited a few moments. The guy tucked the phone between his shoulder and his ear, and pulled out a calculator. Morgan left him reciting figures into the phone and made his way towards the house, sidestepping the clusters of guests and cruising trays of hors d'oeuvres and Roederer Cristal champagne. On the way he saw the newlyweds locked in each other's arms, French kissing before an appreciative audience. Above it all clattered the choppers, like the flies at the wedding cake. Morgan wondered whether the kiss was the real thing or a photo opportunity.

The house was built of redwood, and looked like a transplanted Vermont barn. On the veranda, sheltered from the wind by a wall of glass, a chamber music ensemble was playing for its own enjoyment and that of the catering staff busy setting up tables for the buffet. Morgan was about to ask a waiter the whereabouts of a telephone when he heard his name being called. He saw Niles Kingman, beefy, sandy haired and freckled, like an overgrown Howdy Doody in banker's blue pinstripe, cowboy boots and Stetson, leaning against the bar.

"Long time, no see, Morgan." Kingman saluted him with a squat glass of something golden colored, with ice cubes, and no bubbles.

"Hello, Niles." Morgan went over and shook hands. "Nothing for me," he headed off the approaching bartender.

"I heard you were at this shindig," Kingman said. "Stealing business from us legitimate folk, is that it?"

"I hardly think we're competing for the same market, Niles," Morgan smiled. "It's nice to see you, though. You a friend of the bride or the groom?"

"Pop and I invested a big chunk in Grace Tyler's movie. I guess that got us in good with the California Cooler crowd, right?" Kingman's grin showed an unsettling amount of gleaming white tooth.

"How is your father?"

"Sam? Feistier than ever. We just expanded into

California, and it was all Pop's doing, too. I've been loafing in Europe all summer."

"Lucky you," Morgan said. He stifled the urge to look at his watch. He was anxious to call his truck.

"Yep, we opened up dealerships in San Diego, L.A., and Frisco. Backed it all with a full advertising campaign. Print, radio, TV—the works. Did it all first class, just like we always do.

"Well, good luck. Nice to see you, Niles," Morgan turned to go, but Kingman stopped him.

"Morgan, if we hadn't bumped into one another, I would have looked you up. I have this business proposition I'd like to discuss. I think you'll be interested, seeing as how you're looking to expand."

That spooked the hell out of Morgan. It was true that he had business expansion plans, but they were a closely guarded secret. At least, they were supposed to be.

"Over here, darlin,'" Kingman called out.

Morgan turned. Coming towards them was the knockout redhead in the glen plaid suit.

"Find the little girls' room, okay, darlin'?" Kingman asked. The woman pretended not to hear, and smiled at Morgan, who felt his heartbeat quicken. "Nicole Houel, allow me to introduce Don Morgan," Kingman said.

"I recognized you, from the beginning, Mister Morgan," Nicole Houel confided as she offered Morgan her hand. The caterer could have cut her accent with a knife and served it for dessert. It was aphrodisiac. She flashed a winning smile at Kingman. "Niles, darling, in France, you see, Don Morgan is *still* a celebrity—"

She stopped short, blushing a delicious shade of pink as Kingman chortled, and Morgan feigned despair.

"Oh, please, Mister Morgan! You must forgive me for my stupid blunder!"

She was still holding his hand. She had long, scarlet enameled fingernails. Her eyes were hazel, and she had the lightest scattering of freckles across the bridge of her nose to go along with her red hair.

"Isabelle Huppert," Morgan said.

"Pardon?" She was still holding his hand.

"Who you look like: Isabelle Huppert," Morgan explained.

"I'm flattered, Mister Morgan," she smiled. "But please, you must forgive me—" She was planning to hold his hand forever, he decided. This was not only obvious; it was ordained.

"Of course I forgive you," Morgan said.

She was looking into his eyes as if Kingman weren't there, but then Kingman cleared his throat, and she let go of his hand. Morgan's fingers didn't like it. They wanted to go back where it was warm and soft.

She took hold of Kingman's hand.

"Well," Morgan said, feeling awkward, "I'll let you two get back to the party."

"You going to the Paris Salon, Morgan?" Kingman asked. Morgan nodded. "Me too," Kingman said. "You and I can talk over there."

Morgan smiled at Nicole Houel. "Very nice to have met you, and to know that despite my plummeting star in America, I'm not yet a has-been in France."

She took Kingman's arm as they walked away. Too bad, Morgan thought. It was true, all of the good ones *were* taken . . .

Morgan felt eyes upon him. He turned to see Matt Palmer on the veranda. He was hoisting an attaché case manufactured out of something emerald hued and reptilian, and looking at Morgan in doleful accusation.

"I'm on my way to check on it, Matt."

As if on cue, one of the parking valets approached. "Mister Morgan? I've been looking for you, sir. They told me to tell you the cars are here." He handed Morgan a note.

Morgan sent him off with a buck, and then read the note. It was from one of the crew on the flatrig, assuring Morgan that the merchandise had been delivered in spotless condition. Morgan went over to Palmer.

"They're here?" Palmer demanded excitedly. When Morgan nodded, Palmer exclaimed, "Let's see them!"

They walked around the house, to the circular drive, where the gleaming pair of DeManto 3000 Guerrieri—one black, one white—crouched like panthers. They were low, squat machines, festooned with air scoops and truly evil-looking rear deck wind-spoilers.

Morgan watched, amused, but nevertheless pleased, as Palmer danced around the cars, like a little kid around his presents on Christmas morning.

"Morgan! They're righteous!" Palmer crowed. "They're straight out of Star Wars!"

"More than you can imagine," Morgan nodded. "Keep in mind how quickly you can get yourself into righteous trouble in one of these."

"Are they really fast?" Palmer asked. He set down the attache case, and took a small silver vial from his jacket pocket.

"How's zero to sixty, in under five seconds, while you're still in first gear?"

"*Holy shittt* . . ." Palmer chuckled, unscrewing the vial's lid. "That's faster than a Ferrari, right?"

"These are faster parked than a Ferrari is rolling."

"Seriously, Morgan?"

"Seriously. These two are faster than a Testarossa off the line—top speed, 188 miles per hour, which you'll only use if you plan to commute along the Bonneville Salt Flats."

Palmer tapped some white powder onto the mirror-like surface of the black DeManto's hood, bent low, and snorted it.

"The world's most expensive piece of drug paraphernalia," Morgan said.

Palmer offered him the vial. Morgan declined. Palmer made a wet, sniffling noise, and asked, "Nobody else has cars like these? They're totally gray market?"

Morgan appreciated Palmer's concern. The U.S. version of the DeManto listed for approximately a hundred and twenty grand. Palmer was paying almost double that, per car, in order to have something unique. "Totally, *ultra* gray market," Morgan said. "The authorized export version of this car has fuel injection. What DonSport did was make the carbureted eurocar California street legal." Morgan grinned. "You and Grace should be the only kids on your block with toys like these for some time to come."

Palmer handed Morgan the attaché case. It was heavy, as attaché cases filled with currency will be.

Morgan's business trademark was Cash on Delivery, and it was a damned nuisance. He'd much rather receive a plain, convenient check, but years ago a wise, old film director, for whom Morgan had refurbished a vintage Bentley, had advised him that in this corner of the world, image was everything. The cagey director had been right. By demanding cash on the line, Morgan was giving his clients a melodramatic thrill concerning their purchases, a sense that they were getting something really hot.

"Morgan," Palmer called. He was combing his pompadour by his reflection in the black Guerrieri's hood. "That attaché cost three grand, but I want you to have it as a gift."

"That's very kind of you," Morgan politely replied.

They always gave him the attaché case as a gift, and he, in turn, distributed them to his employees at DonSport. Morgan had received three of these particular lizard and gold cases from clients, just this month. Bijan must have been having a clearance sale.

Grace's album was blaring from somewhere on the ocean side of the house. Morgan wondered what the chamber music ensemble was thinking; he thought Grace had a singing voice like Betty Boop on Spanish fly. This particular song—"Candy and Tattoos"—had been the biggest of the several hits off the album. The radio stations had played it endlessly.

9

"The keys are in the ignitions," Morgan told Palmer. "Manuals translated into English are in the glove compartments, but what I advise is for you to call DonSport when you're ready, and I'll send one of my people around to instruct you and Grace—"

"Yeah, sure, Morgan," Palmer cut him off. "About Grace, and what happened a little while ago . . . I hope you didn't get the wrong idea. I mean, she was just kidding, you know?"

Morgan looked at Palmer, and could almost see himself, dauntless and cocky, some fifteen years ago. Back then, he'd believed that staying honest was what helped him to win, on the race track and in life. Eventually he'd found out that winning is just as much a matter of luck as it is skill or honesty, and that sooner or later, luck runs out.

"Nothing happened, Matt, except that your new bride was feeling a little too good."

"Well, I just wanted you to know, I don't blame *you*," Palmer said quietly, and then he brightened. "Anyway," he patted the white DeManto's hood. "Wait 'til she sees this."

"Call DonSport if you have any problems, Matt," Morgan said.

"You going Morgan?" Palmer asked, surprised. "Why not stick around? The party's just getting started . . ."

"Matt, take care of yourself, *and* your wife."

"What? Yeah, sure, Morgan."

Morgan walked over to the parking valets standing nearby. "The pine green 635," he told the nearest one.

"You know how many BMW 635s I've got parked, mister?"

"It's the convertible."

"The what?" The kid looked blank, then incredulous.

"*I* saw it," one of the others piped up. "I'll get it for you, sir."

The kid was back in under two minutes with the car.

"I'm a BMW freak," the kid said as Morgan tipped him. "I've restored half a dozen 2002s. Where do you get a car like this? I mean, you just can't walk into a dealship and *buy* it, can you?"

"What you do is have the hard-top sawed off and a soft-top installed."

The kid looked like he was ready to come. "I'd *love* to do that kind of work," he sighed.

Morgan looked at him a moment, and then quietly said, "I know." He took a business card out of his billfold and handed it to the kid. "Call for an appointment to see Martin Robbins. If you're any good—and Mister Robbins will know if you are—you *can* do this kind of work."

The kid looked at the name on the card, and then back at Morgan. "You him, sir? Damn! My dad told me about you!"

Morgan winced.

"How delightful, I adore convertibles."

It was Nicole Houel. She had a black, saddlebag styled, Porsche Design carryall slung over her shoulder. "Mister Morgan, if it is not too much trouble, I wonder if I might have a ride back to San Francisco?"

"Um, what about Niles?" Morgan asked as he stowed the attaché case in the BMW's trunk.

She cocked her head. "What about him, Mister Morgan?"

Okay, fine, Morgan thought. "I'd adore taking you for a ride, Ms. Houel."

The valets bumped into each other scurrying to open the door for her as she threw her bag into the convertible's back seat.

2

THEY DROVE NORTH on State One along the Monterey coastline, enjoying the Oriental-looking landscape of wind-wracked cypresses, slate-hued, crashing waves, and barren, rocky islands teeming with comorants and seals. Morgan was in no hurry, and Nicole had a camera and wanted to use it, so they stopped often. The sun began to sink, and the late afternoon turned blustery. Nicole insisted that Morgan keep the top down on the BMW. She'd long ago stowed her hat in deference to the wind. Her fuzzy halo of hair gleamed like copper as the light turned orange, and then the color of old gold. She looked magnificent.

It was getting dark as they rejoined State One, but it was still warm enough to keep the convertible's top down. Morgan turned on his lights, kept an eye on his radar detector, and let the BMW unwind. For a moment he felt that old elation as the sudden acceleration pressed him back against the leather bucket seat. Quickly, though, the elation faded away.

"You drive very fast," Nicole said, sounding more amused than concerned.

"I can slow down if you'd feel more comfortable?" Morgan offered as he slid past the slower moving traffic.

"Please enjoy yourself."

Morgan sighed. "For me driving is just a way to get from one place to another."

"You don't enjoy driving?"

"It's no big deal."

Nicole was watching the speedometer. "It is hard to believe we are going so fast, the ride is so smooth and steady . . ."

"Jackie Stewart says that the key to effective driving is to anticipate problems, and keep a constant, steady pace. He believes that the most successful competition drivers don't even get noticed until they win."

"Were you as good as Jackie Stewart, Mister Morgan?"

"No." He thought about it. "I might have been."

She was waiting, clearly expecting him to say more. She'd have a long wait.

"But you were good?" she finally asked.

"Yes."

"Do you ever get the urge to get back on a track?"

"No."

She chuckled. "Mister Morgan, would you like me to change the subject?"

"Yes." Morgan was grateful that she was willing to let it alone.

"I see, a man of few words, like your American cowboys. Very well, consider the subject changed." She twisted around to reach her bag on the back seat. "You have spent so much time in Europe, Mister Morgan. Do you have any French?"

Morgan shrugged. "What I had was an entourage to speak for me when necessary, but most of the people I mixed with spoke English. Anyway, I guess I picked up a little menu French, and car Italian." Morgan smiled. "And bedroom German . . ."

"Pardon?"

"Never mind. Private joke, and not a very funny one, at that." He watched as she pawed through her bag. "Just how much junk have you got stowed in that thing?" he asked as she pulled out a bulky, cotton cardigan sweater, a small tape recorder, and a package of Pall Malls.

"As a journalist I need the tools of my trade close at

13

hand." She took off her suit coat, stowed it in her bag, and put on the sweater. Then she extracted a cigarette, and tapped its unfiltered end on her thumb nail. "Can I smoke?"

"I don't know, we'll see."

"Pardon?"

"Just another old joke. We Americans are chock full of them. So you're a journalist? Who do you write for?"

"I free-lance," she explained, "for a number of newspapers and magazines in France."

"Is that why you were at the wedding, to do a story on Matt and Grace?" Morgan asked.

"No, but is that what you really want to know?"

"Hmm?"

"I think what you really want to know is what I was doing there with Niles Kingman, yes, Mister Morgan?"

"It's on my mind," Morgan smiled. "And please call me Don, or Morgan. Anything but Mister. After that wedding I feel old enough already."

"But what how old could you be? No more than forty?"

"A smidgen more," Morgan said wistfully. "It must be the tie that dates me. Or maybe my socks . . ."

"Your socks?"

"I wear them."

"I think you look splendid," she assured him. "And please call me Nicole—" She paused as a small, matte black box mounted on the center console near the cellular phone, hummed, then a red light on the thing began to flash.

"Car phone answering machine," Morgan explained.

"Ah, America," Nicole laughed. "Land of gadgets! You may take your call."

"Don't want to," Morgan replied. "I'm talking to you, now."

"Morgan, I'm intrigued. Most Americans are slaves to their telephones. "Tell me, do you sometimes not answer your telephone at home?"

14

"My home number's unlisted. About six people in the world know it, and I change it every few months, just to keep it that way. I can be reached in the car, or at work. That's enough."

She smiled. "You *are* a cowboy."

"You were telling me about yourself, and Niles."

"We are very good friends. We met in Paris. Niles was vacationing, and I was just beginning a series of articles for *Le Monde* on world-class entrepreneurs. I interviewed Niles for my series. When he ran into you at the party, and it turned out you were friends, it occurred to me that it would be useful to interview you about Niles and his father in order to get another perspective on them."

"I'm disappointed. You aren't interested in me?"

"I could be," she laughed lightly. "But right now I am after Niles."

She said that last bit oddly, Morgan thought. As if it were her turn to make a private joke. "So, this ride is a business trip?"

Morgan watched her switch on her tape recorder. "I guess it's a business trip. Well, let's see what I can tell you about Kingman and Son . . . Some time ago, as you might recall, Chrysler Corporation was in deep, financial trouble, and looking for loans from the government. They weren't going to get those loans, until Sam Kingman telephoned the senators he has in his pocket."

"You see?" Nicole smiled. "Niles told me nothing of this. I had no idea his father was that powerful."

Sam owns fifty or so assorted American and Japanese dealerships, across the country. Through every one of those dealerships he contributes to Congressional campaigns. That translates into a lot of influence in Washington. His company went public a few years ago. He's what's called a mega-dealer. I suppose his closest European counterpart would be Helmut Becker."

"Who?"

"Helmut Becker?" *For a journalist writing about*

European and American entrepreneurs, you certainly haven't done much homework, Morgan thought. "Becker runs a company in Düsseldorf, called Auto-Becker. It imports, sells, and distributes seventeen different car lines."

"Oh, yes, of course," she nodded impatiently. "But what can you tell me about Niles?"

"First off, there's a pretty good seafood place in Pescadero, if you're hungry?"

"I'm fine. I ate so much at the wedding."

Morgan nodded. "About Niles, then. I don't really know how to put this. Niles is not exactly what you'd call a chip off the old block. I mean, his father is still out there working eighteen hour days, but Niles—"

"He's a fuck-off—Yes, Morgan?"

"Fuck-off, fuck-up, however you want to put it," Morgan chuckled. "It looks like you already know everything there is to know about Niles. Please don't quote me, but I doubt that Niles would be able to keep the family business intact without his father."

"What about his gambling?" she asked.

"What?"

"Come now, Morgan, you must have heard that Niles has run up substantial gambling debts in certain private London clubs?"

"Why would I know that?"

"But you are close friends, no?"

"No. Niles and I are more business acquaintances than friends, Nicole."

"I see . . ."

"I'm very sorry if you somehow got the idea that I was close to Niles."

"Well, perhaps you will be," she replied brightly.

San Francisco, lit up, shrouded in fog, glowed with ghostly luminescence as they drove along the Bayshore Freeway, past the airport, towards the heart of the city. Nicole, bundled up in her sweater, her tape recorder stowed away, was enjoying the soft night, and the ride, as Morgan expertly weaved the snarling BMW through the heavy traffic.

"Where are you staying?" he asked.

"The Fairmont." She hesitated. "I don't want to put you to any trouble—"

"Oh, it's no trouble," Morgan said. "I live in the Nob Hill area. My condo's just a few blocks away from the Fairmont."

"I'm flying to London tomorrow morning." She looked at him out of the corners of her eyes. "But I really don't want to spend my last night in your country alone in my hotel room. Do you suppose we could go to your apartment for a drink?"

"I thought this was business," Morgan pretended to complain.

"This is called mixing business with pleasure."

Morgan left the freeway to join the traffic shuffling along Sacramento Street. He drove past the manicured greenery of Huntington Park, and then turned right, onto his street lined with baroque, Crayola-colored townhouses, presided over by the high tower of his ultramodern condo building. Anywhere else in America the clashing architecture would jar, but it all seemed to fit together in wacky harmony here in the City by the Bay.

He pulled into his building's circular driveway, and used a magnetic strip card to open the gate to the underground garage. He parked the BMW, then grabbed his overnighter and the cash-laden attaché case. He noticed that Nicole was taking her own overnighter upstairs.

He wondered how he felt about that. It had taken him a long time to come to the conclusion that it was all right for a guy to have something other than the automatic response to the opportunity of going to bed with a woman. He led her to the elevators, which they took up to Morgan's penthouse. He unlocked his door and invited her in.

"A very American apartment," Nicole smiled, as

Morgan showed her around. The apartment was spacious and airy, with its minimum of furniture crafted of oak and mocha glove leather. There was track lighting, and a fireplace framed in gray slate. The walls were finished in rough stucco, and whitewashed. There was lots of oak trim, and oak floors, polished to a high, honey sheen, and dotted with brightly colored wool Dhurrie rugs.

He led her out through the French doors, to the wraparound terrace and its sweeping views of Russian Hill. The lights of the North Beach waterfront glimmered in the distance.

"Your home is very elegant," Nicole murmured, standing close to him on the dark terrace. "The way you are elegant, in the American style. It is not European elegance, but perhaps that is why I am attracted to it, and to you, so very much."

Morgan kissed her. She smelled like some brand of soap he couldn't place, and like tobacco, and a bit like the salty night. She felt soft and very warm beneath her cotton sweater.

She briefly nibbled at his lower lip before she pulled away. Morgan felt weak.

"Good thing there's a railing," he murmured.

"Or you would be head over heels?"

Morgan flinched. She'd said it in a shitty kind of way; sort of cynical. It pissed him off. It also scared him a little. She was running a little too hot and cold. Suddenly he realized what was really spooking him. She was a lot like Ilsa.

"Come inside. You've got a drink coming," Morgan said. She was leaning forward, resting her elbows on the railing. The bulky sweater was bunched up around her waist and her skirt was stretched tight; she was promoting the hell out of her pornographic derrière.

"I hear anger in your voice. Why are you angry?"

No longer a bitch, but a little French girl, Morgan thought. *Poor,* little French girl . . . Yes, she was spooky as hell. And Morgan liked it.

"Come inside," he told her.

"But why?"

Her hair was a riotous mass of curls in the breeze blowing off of the bay, and her lips looked slightly swollen.

"Come inside, before I fuck your brains out right here on the cement," Morgan growled, then turned and went back into the apartment. He sat down on the couch and waited. It was a stupid game, a childish test of wills, but Morgan knew her type; the game had to be played before they could get anywhere. The living room creaked with silence. He got up and took Palmer's attaché case into the kitchen, stashing it in the wall safe hidden behind a swingout shelf unit in the pantry. He went back into the living room. She was still out on the terrace. He strode over to the fireplace, piled up some kindling and a few small sticks, and lit a fire.

She came in and stood beside him while he was fiddling with the fire. She was wearing gray high heels, he noticed, and gray nylons with a subtle floral pattern woven into them. Her toe began tapping impatiently. "White wine would be fine," she said.

Morgan threw a couple of logs on the fire, and went into the kitchen, where he checked the whites he had chilled. He selected a half bottle of a Puligny-Montrachet. He pulled the cork, took down two wine glasses, filled one with apple juice from the fridge, put everything on a tray and brought it into the living room. Nicole, looking like a college kid with her touseled hair and bulky sweater, was curled up on the rug by the fireplace, smoking a Pall Mall, and flicking her ashes into the flames.

"In the spirit of renewed international cooperation," Morgan said, setting the tray on a nearby end table, and showing her the wine label. He poured her some, and settled down beside her on the rug.

"What are you drinking?" she asked, taking off her sweater.

"Apple juice."

"You don't drink?"

"Oh, I'm a splendid drinker. It's *stopping* that's my problem."

"You mean you are an ex-alcoholic?"

"No, I mean I'm an alcoholic, but I *am* an ex-drinker."

"For how long?"

"You mean, since I've had a drink? About nine years—" *and three months, two weeks, four days, eight hours and counting.* He wondered why he was talking about it. It was no secret, but he rarely talked about it.

"But Morgan, you have wine in your apartment, and I see a liquor cabinet."

"I have friends who like to drink," he said simply.

She nodded, and took a sip of her wine. "May I say that it is very good?"

Morgan laughed. "Yes, you may. And please enjoy it."

"I have a little coke that Niles gave me. Would you care for it?"

Morgan made a face. "No thanks. That stuff is poison."

Nicole sighed, sounding sadly amused. "Oh, Morgan . . . Are you again speaking from personal experience?"

"In a way. I was close to someone who couldn't handle it. But that's a long story."

She took another sip of wine, watching him over the rim of the glass. "Morgan, would you please take me to bed? I would very much like to see what you *do* indulge in."

What happened was, she took *him* to bed. In the bedroom she undressed herself, which Morgan kind of liked. After all, whatever this was—and Morgan wanted it—it was not romance.

It's certainly going to be exercise, Morgan thought as she stood before him, a splendid redhead in a pair of sky blue, silk bikini pants. He went over and fetched her. Her cleavage made an enthralling, liquid sound as her hardened nipples rubbed against his bare chest.

They tumbled onto Morgan's big bed and kissed a while, taking their time, being tentative, exploring the ways their bodies might fit together. A mournful fog horn on the bay played counterpoint to the whispery rustling of the sheets, and their gasps as they touched each other's intimate places for the first time. She was as deft as a surgeon with her scarlet enameled, mandarin fingernails. Nerve endings between Morgan's legs began tap dancing beneath her touch. He tried to slide off her bikini pants.

"Tear them," she said.

He did. A tattered strip of lacy silk remained draped around her flat belly above the flaring curves of her hips.

When he entered her she flexed her fingers into claws to lightly furrow his back. She hissed something in French. Her spine arched and her hips bucked. Her head, her hair fanning scarlet against the white pillow, began to thrash from side to side.

This bitch is acting, Morgan thought. "Stop it!" The harshness in his own voice surprised him.

She froze. Instantly. She gave him a hazel-eyed stare a Siamese cat would have killed for. There must have been something scary in his own eyes, because she said, "Please . . ." and there was no bullshit left in her, none at all.

"At least now we're on the same side," Morgan said, gently this time. He still couldn't figure her out. Out in the world, in her designer clothes, she was formidable, but in bed—with her dragon lady act put aside—she was too vulnerable a creature with which to do battle. He stopped fucking her and started to make love. She began to relax, closing her eyes for a time, then suddenly popping them open, as if she were surprised he was still there.

"It will be too long for you," she said sadly.

"Honey, a guy who has the will power to lay off the booze for nine years ain't about to come too soon—"

She hugged him then, and closed her eyes again, and went away to wherever it was she had to go to make it happen. At the last possible instant, she made the effort—he *knew* she did—to come back to him. And Morgan was there for her. When he came it felt fine; no more, no less. What pleased him more was the way she held him close, murmuring something. It, too, was in French, but it sounded lots kinder than what she'd said that first time around.

Eventually she slid out from under him, got out of bed, and went jiggly-wiggly into the living room, coming back with her wine and cigarettes. She was about to light up when she paused, and said, "Morgan, this is your bedroom, and you don't smoke, can I?"

"We now know the answer is yes."

It took her a second to work out the English language pun on the word "smoke." "Now I get the joke!" she laughed, curling up beside him. "I need to tell you about what happened, why I—"

Morgan put a finger to her lips. She looked down at him, and all at once her expression went sad. "You are always in control? You never let loose?"

There was nothing to say to that, so he said the best thing he could think of. "Let's try smoking again."

3

MORGAN WOKE A little before dawn. Outside it was still dark, but they'd fallen asleep with the bedside lamp on. Nicole was out of it, snoring softly.

Go back to sleep, he thought, but instead he folded his arms behind his head, stared up at the ceiling, and brooded about Niles Kingman. That Kingman had somehow learned about his plans to expand troubled him, but more unsettling was the realization that someone in Morgan's inner circle, someone he *trusted*, had leaked that information. . . . Well, he couldn't do anything about that until tomorrow.

Morgan sighed. It wasn't only his worries about Kingman that were keeping him awake. He'd been dreaming of Ilsa. He guessed that attending the wedding, and being with Nicole, had stirred up the memories, or maybe it was just that there really were ghosts—but where they prowled was the attic of the mind, not some old haunted house.

Damn, but it was hard to dream of Ilsa and then have to wake up! It was like being forced to suffer the pain of losing her all over again.

In his dreams Ilsa wasn't drawn and haggard, and her arms were not a festered mass of needle tracks. In his dreams Ilsa looked the way she did on the day he'd first laid eyes on her.

But inevitably the dream had to end. "Life goes on." So the saying went, but for Morgan, life never really did go on after Ilsa. . . .

Lying there, with Nicole sleeping beside him, Morgan was filled with a wistful longing for the past, when he'd gone from pauper to prince, and married the princess.

When he finished his Army hitch in '65, his parents wanted him to return to high school to get his diploma, but Morgan knew what he wanted: to be a pro stock car race driver. For that you didn't need the kind of education they taught in classrooms. He was great behind the wheel; not so hot tinkering underneath the hood, but he knew enough to get a job at a garage in his hometown of Fiskboro, Massachusetts, fifteen miles south of Boston. Morgan eventually plunked down a couple of hundred on a dilapidated '59 Ford Galaxie. It came free of charge with peeling "STP" and "Champion Spark Plugs" decals on the rear windows, and a scab of rust all along the fender wells. Its 292 cubic inch V-8 engine burned a couple of quarts of oil a week, but you stomped that mother and she moved out.

He was a gawky looking kid. He favored white T-shirts and pegged jeans tucked into black engineer's boots. He had a faint moustache and an Elvis inspired duck's ass haircut tall enough to leave Vitalis skid marks on the Galaxie's frayed headliner. He raced on dirt tracks hidden out in the boondocks, and the larger paved tracks of New England, like Massachusetts' Seekonk Speedway and Thunder Road in Vermont. He won most every race he entered, but first place usually paid only fifty or a hundred bucks, and he was going through tires, brake pads, and clutches like they were toilet paper, so he was always in the hole.

He was up at Quarry Speedway, in Vermont, where he took first place in a Night Owls' Funny Car Free For All, when he met Lee Thomas. Morgan and some friends were loading the Galaxie up onto the flatbed he'd borrowed from the garage where he worked, and celebrating Morgan's win by passing around a fifth of Canadian Club, when Thomas showed up.

"A word with you, boyo." The guy's thick Irish brogue said it all about where he'd come from. "By the way, me heartiest congrats on your win."

"Thanks." Morgan didn't know who this guy was, but a sixth sense told him that he was *someone*. The guy was in his late thirties, with a Mitch Miller beard, and thick brown hair, worn long, in a kind of soupbowl haircut, like Moe from the Stooges, or those Beatles. He wore a white, fisherman's turtleneck sweater, a burgundy leather jacket, sharkskin slacks, and shiny burgundy boots that zipped up the side.

"Can we talk in private?" the guy asked, sounding like Barry Fitzgerald. "Take a little walk with me, boyo."

Morgan nodded. "Be right back," Morgan promised his friends, but somehow he knew he wouldn't.

"My name's Lee Thomas. Have you ever heard of me?" They'd gone a few paces, leaving Morgan's friends in the shadows.

"Can't say that I have, Mister."

Thomas chuckled. "I race on the Grand Prix circuit, sponsored by DeManto. You have heard of them, I assume."

Morgan laughed. "They make those fancy Italian sports cars that cost a mint. Who *hasn't* heard of them. If you drive Formula One, you must be here for the big race at Watkins Glen next week."

Thomas nodded. "While my crew is toying with my racer I thought I'd have a holiday. I heard about this race, and thought I'd come to see how this stock car thing is done."

They were walking along the stretch of grandstand paralleling the straightaway, just before the finish line. The stands were empty now. The last, loitering members of the crowd were shuffling out through the exit gates. The concession stands were shutting down, while the big, furry Vermont moths were enjoying one final, frenzied, suicide dance around the high, hissing floodlights.

"I've got a team to back me up, a team of mechanics, to be sure, but also a number of apprentice drivers. DeManto pays them, but I pick them." Thomas stopped and put both hands on Morgan's shoulders. "I pick *you,* boyo. You've got the makings of something quite extraordinary behind the wheel, and I want to own it." He smiled. "For as long as possible, at any rate. I want you to join my team."

"Holy shit, Mister Thomas. You mean like go to Europe?" Morgan blushed. He was sounding stupid. Like Maynard on "Dobie Gillis."

Thomas laughed. "Don't worry, you won't have to swim there."

"Holy shit—I mean, I don't believe it. I don't know what to say."

"Say yes." Thomas shrugged. "Why not? You're not married, are you? Or is it the thought of leaving behind your girlfriend that's troubling you?"

Morgan shook his head. He'd never even slept with a girl. Oh, sure, lots of them were available during his hitch in the Army, but they weren't the type to turn him on. There were some real nice girls back home in Fiskboro, but with his nights and weekends taken up with racing there wasn't any time for dating. Anyway, you needed money to take a girl out, and all of Morgan's cash went toward the upkeep of his car. "For how long? I mean is this a permanent job you're offering me?"

"It's a competition, boyo. There's a number of Young Turks on me team. As we go along we winnow 'em out. I promise you that you'll always have a ticket home, but beyond that I make no promises." Thomas took a folded sheet of paper out of his pocket and handed it to Morgan. "You come to Watkins Glen a week from tomorrow, if you have a mind to. You show that note to the gatekeeper, and they'll give you a badge that'll get you pitside. My crew will know that you might be coming."

Morgan unfolded the paper. Inside was a hundred dollar bill. "Mister, I can't take this."

"Sure you can. For your travel expenses to Watkins Glen. You can't use tonight's winnings for that, it wouldn't be fair to your mates." Thomas shook hands with Morgan. "A week from Sunday, then. And if not, good luck to you."

Morgan watched him walk away, then returned to the flat rig. He made up some story for his buddies, because he wasn't yet ready to discuss what the Irishman had said. They drove all through the night, arriving back in Fiskboro around ten on Sunday morning. Morgan made the trip curled up on the back seat of the Galaxie. He tried to doze, but it was impossible. He was still too full of the race, and Lee Thomas's fantastic offer.

All that week Morgan spent his nights at the library, foraging through the newspaper stacks, reading up on Formula One racing, and on Lee Thomas.

On Thursday he told his boss at the garage he wasn't going to be in the next day. By dawn Friday morning, equipped with road maps, a case of motor oil, half a dozen assorted Drake's Cakes, a six pack of Royal Crown Cola, and a box of NoDoz, Morgan was on the road to Watkins Glen. He took it slow, scared that the Galaxie would conk out. He arrived late that night, only to be told by a state cop that there wasn't a vacant motel room within a hundred miles. So Morgan spent a long, cold, miserable night wrapped up in his bench warmer in the back seat of his car. Early Sunday morning he presented his note to a gatekeeper, who directed Morgan to a trailer where he was issued a cardboard tag to wear around his neck. He wandered around the bustling Watkins Glen facility until he found his way to the DeManto pit. There he saw Thomas, suited up in his racing gear, who gave him a cursory nod. Morgan hung back, knowing a driver needed to be by himself for those last few minutes before a race.

27

Thomas went to climb into his car, and the mechanics who'd been swarming like ants over the thing, all stood away.

Morgan stared at it. He stared at that car. The Formula One DeManto was a single seat, open cockpit torpedo. It didn't even look like a car; it lacked fenders, lights, doors, even a windshield; with its tall, fat, black tires, and huge, rear mounted engine, it looked like a speedboat on waterwings. And it was fire engine red: *DeManto red.* That special hue forged of flame and blood was as much a part of the Italian manufacturer's trademark as the proud hood badge depicting a black unicorn, rampant, upon a gray shield.

All around the track engines were bellowing to life. Lee Thomas started his own engine. If the other cars sounded like bulls, or lions, the DeManto sounded panther shrill, as high-strung, and as implacably fierce.

Thomas moved his car out onto the track. Morgan, watching, thought that he would gladly commit murder to be behind the wheel—*to be in command of that car.*

The race began, and from that moment on Morgan knew exactly what he was going to do.

Sunday night Morgan drove home. He was dizzy from lack of sleep, but wired and giddy over his future. It was late Monday morning by the time he got back to Fiskboro. He drove straight to the garage, where he quit his job. He went home, explained it all as best he could to his parents, and then signed over to them the Galaxie's pink slip.

He took the train from Boston to New York City, where he linked up with the Thomas/DeManto team at the airport. The entourage included seven mechanics; three apprentice drivers; Thomas, his wife, and their three little girls; the DeManto Formula One and a back-up car; a spare parts, tires, and tools trailer; and now Morgan, himself.

"Welcome to the circus," Thomas grinned that evening, halfway across the Atlantic during the first airplane ride of Morgan's life. "Here's a present for you, boyo," Thomas said, handing Morgan a jacket. "Try and get some sleep. We'll be in London in a few hours." He went off to his own seat.

He unfolded the jacket that Thomas had given him. It was cut from some silvery material, and emblazoned on the breast pocket, the right sleeve, and on the back, bigger than life, was the DeManto prancing unicorn.

It was 1966. Morgan was 19 years old. He was on the team.

The next year was the happiest in Morgan's life. Grand Prixes were held in the most exotic and glamorous cities of the world, and everywhere the teams visited, they were wined and dined and treated like royalty. At his first race, the Gran Premio de España, held in Barcelona, Thomas let him take the Formula One on a test run around the track.

"Was it all you'd thought it would be, Donnie?" Thomas asked him as Morgan guided the car back into the pit.

"Better, Lee," Morgan breathed. "Better than I thought *anything* could be."

"Well, now you're no longer a virgin," Thomas said, and the others laughed.

Half right, Morgan thought to himself. That night, wandering the streets of Barcelona, he found a pretty little waitress in a tapas bar. She had raven black hair and big brown eyes like a puppy dog, and spoke enough English to understand what Morgan was getting at. She had a room nearby. She took his virginity, and he gave her his DeManto jacket, which was what she'd been into all along. Walking back to the hotel Morgan thought to himself that it definitely beat jacking off, but not by a hell of a lot. Next morning at the hotel he got himself another team jacket. The circus carried along dozens; the guys were always trading them for *something*.

DeManto wasn't paying him very much, but his room

and board were taken care of, so whatever cash he had he could blow. In London and in Paris he bought clothes, and even threw away his Vitalis, getting his hair cut like Lee Thomas'. Morgan still preferred Elvis to the Yardbirds, but he kept that to himself. Every night, in a different hotel dining room or restaurant, Thomas and the others taught Morgan about food and wine. When Thomas found out Morgan had never finished high school he jotted down a few books Morgan might want to read. Morgan devoured them, more to impress his idol than to actually learn anything, but the learning came, nevertheless.

Once Morgan asked Thomas if he ought to learn French or Italian. "Not needed, Donnie," Thomas replied. "If the French and Italians and whatnot want to talk to you, they'll find a way. If they don't, they'll pretend they can't understand you, no matter how good you get at their jabber."

Morgan was attracting girls at every stop. Birds were what Lee Thomas called them. They were young, and pretty, and willing to do anything with any guy who could get them within touching distance of a Formula One. Morgan thought that maybe the reason fucking wasn't a big deal to him yet was because it was an acquired taste, like port. So he practiced fucking the same way he practiced driving: with total dedication and concentration. Actually, the two activities seemed to have a lot in common.

He was sure that he was doing it right. The birds carried on about it so! Sometimes they even wanted him to fuck them again instead of going for a spin in the car, and that was as high an endorsement as they could give. To Morgan it felt good, just like it had that first time in Barcelona, but he still enjoyed driving more.

In Germany, during the week prior to the Nüburgring run, there was some mechanical trouble with the Formula One. Concerned about it, Lee Thomas backed out of a publicity photo session in Frankfurt that he had committed to on behalf of the West German DeManto distributorship. The publicist quickly looked over the apprentice drivers, and picked Morgan as Thomas' stand-in. Nothing to it, the publicist assured a very nervous Morgan as they journeyed from out of the shadows of the Eifel Mountains. Morgan would just pose in his racing jacket alongside a line-up of DeManto vehicles.

Oh, and there would be a model taking part in the photo session . . .

She wore white, knee-high boots, black, fishnet stockings, a gold, leather miniskirt, and a black turtleneck sweater. She was tall, almost as tall as Morgan. She had brown eyes the color and shape of almonds, and blonde hair, cut like Cleopatra's. The stylist at the shoot brushed it smooth and flat so that when she tossed her head it shimmered and moved like the finest chain link forged from platinum.

Her name was Ilsa Wolff. Her German accented English gave Morgan a hard-on. Once, when she bent over to tug at her boot, her miniskirt rode up and Morgan caught a glimpse of white thigh and black garter belt. The peek gave him a worse hard-on. The photographer kept yelling at Morgan—Thomas had been right, when they wanted to talk to you, they spoke English—to look at the cars, or the camera, or the sky, or anything, but to stop looking at Ilsa.

Ilsa giggled, and asked why he was so distracted? Morgan blushed furiously. His mouth was bone dry, and he was sure he was going to faint. He plaintively told her, "I can't stop looking at you . . . you're so beautiful."

"You are such a sweet boy," she laughed gaily, kissing him lightly on the lips.

"Gotchya—"

Startled, Morgan jumped back.

"Groovy. Catch you both, later," the photographer added as he packed away his camera equipment.

31

When Morgan turned back, Ilsa had already disappeared.

A few minutes later he was on his way back to the circus. He knew that in a few days the race would be over, the circus would leave Germany, and he would never see Ilsa Wolff again. He thought about writing to her, but what would be the point? They'd spent an hour together; she had probably already forgotten him. He told himself to put Ilsa Wolff out of his mind.

And he did, for days at a stretch, as the circus meandered the Grand Prix circuit to Monaco, France, the Netherlands, Britain, Austria, and Portugal. But now, whenever he took the birds to bed, Ilsa's image would come unbidden, and Morgan began to comprehend just what it was about sex he was missing. He had never been in love, until now.

During a break in the Grand Prix schedule the Thomas circus returned to Italy, and the DeManto factory grounds outside of Modena, a few kilometers from the factories of DeManto's chief rival, Ferrari. Years ago, Professor Erberto DeManto and Enzo Ferrari had worked side by side as mechanics for Alfa-Romeo, then settled here to become "friendly" competitors, and ultimately, automotive legends. Their presence had made the region a mecca for sports car enthusiasts.

Morgan spent his days at the DeManto grounds refining his driving and helping the mechanics work on the Formula One. The other apprentice drivers made fun of him for "getting his hands dirty," but Morgan felt that the more he knew about the DeManto, the better driver he'd be.

He was in the garage when Lee Thomas came to talk with him.

"Donnie, take a walk with me," Thomas said.

Morgan, wiping the grease from his hands, thought back to how Thomas had come into his life with just those same words. Back then he'd felt that something momentous was about to happen, and he'd been right. He knew something momentous was about to happen now.

Thomas was quiet and unusually serious as they left the garage. Morgan followed him into the labyrinthine, overgrown gardens surrounding the ivy covered, stone castle that was home to both Professor DeManto and his company's offices. It was an overcast day, and there was a breeze blowing, sending scarlet and yellow leaves swirling against the old, eroded statuary of angels and devils that played hide-and-seek among the trees. Thomas told Morgan to take a seat beside him on a marble bench.

"Donnie, I've been wondering," Thomas began. "When were you planning on going back home to America?"

Morgan freaked. *Oh, God, he said it was a competition; I've lost, and he's going to give me my ticket home.* He took a deep breath. "Lee, as far as I'm concerned, the circus and DeManto are my home."

Thomas nodded. "That's what I was hoping to hear. You see, I've got a bit of a proposition to make. The automobile manufacturers have a championship series of races of their own, the Championnat Internationale de Marques. Old man DeManto has a new car he wants to put up against the best the Krauts, and whatnot, have to offer. He calls it a Rivendicatore GTA-999." He lowered his voice. "That's wop talk for Vindicator."

Morgan nodded. "You want me to stick around to test drive it, Lee?"

Thomas smiled. "More than that, Donnie. The manufacturers' races are endurance events. Some are six hours long, and others, at Le Mans and Daytona Beach go twenty-four hours. There must be at least two drivers on each team. I've talked it over with the Professor. He's given me his blessing to make you my relief driver.

33

Morgan stared at Thomas, trying to comprehend what the Irishman had just said. "You mean," he began in a mouse small voice, "that I'm going to get to drive for DeManto, in a real race?"

"As real as it gets, boyo," Thomas laughed.

"But Lee, I never have—driven in a race, I mean—since joining up with you."

"But you've been driving a hell of a lot; I've been watching you. You're better than my other apprentices, even though they've been around longer, but what really tips the scales in your favor is that you're a Yank. There's only a handful of you Americans on the Grand Prix and Manufacturers' circuits. Both the Professor and I agree that if we do well together as a team it'll mean a lot of publicity for DeManto's new car." Thomas nudged Morgan's ribs. "Won't that make a certain Italian gent in the same line of work as our Professor grit his teeth, Donnie?"

Morgan's first race was to be in Germany, back at Nüburgring in the Eifel Mountains, near the German/Belgian border. On impulse Morgan decided to telephone Ilsa Wolff to give her the news that he'd be back in Germany in a few weeks, and ask her if she would come watch his first race. He tracked her down with the help of the DeManto publicist. When he heard her voice over the phone Morgan's knees went weak. He managed to stammer out who he was, and Ilsa said she remembered him. She congratulated him on his promotion, and said that she would very much like to come see him drive.

Morgan hung up, giddy. It was hard to say what he looked forward to more: the race, or the opportunity to be with Ilsa. The time passed slowly. Morgan practiced his driving by day, and dreamt of Ilsa at night. He couldn't stop thinking about her during the plane ride to Germany the week before the race, but upon his arrival at the hotel there was a telegram waiting for him at the front desk. It was from Ilsa, apologizing, but an extended photo shoot had come up at the last instant. . . .

That night he and Thomas went out. Morgan got drunk, and at some point he took the scrap of paper with Ilsa's telephone number out of his wallet, crumpled it up, and set fire to it in an ashtray. Thomas asked him what it was. Morgan, watching the scrap curl in the little match flame, and then crumple to ash, said it was nothing at all.

The day of the race, Thomas took the first and third driving stints; Morgan spelled him for the middle stint. The race was not a triumph for either DeManto or Morgan, who was rusty behind the wheel. It had been over a year since he'd competed with other drivers. The big, blood-red DeManto 999 was just too much car for him that day, and he was thrown by the fact that the course was crowded with everything from little Fiats to Chevy Corvettes. The purpose of the mixed bag of cars was to provide an opportunity for every auto manufacturer in the world to win a *first-in-class* finish that they could later exploit in advertising. For Morgan it was like being in rush hour traffic on a serpentine, narrow turnpike, except that this rush hour was being conducted at speeds up to 200 mph, and the only rule of the road was "go fast and win."

To top it all off, he couldn't concentrate. He kept fantasizing that Ilsa Wolff was out there, somewhere, cheering him on.

His driving stint over, Morgan guided the rumbling DeManto prototype into the pit area.

"Lee, I'm sorry I stroked it," Morgan said, near tears as he climbed out of the car.

"Don't worry, Donnie," Thomas said lightly as the pit crew did their frenzied jitterbug around the smoking 999. "I expected as much your first time out. I'm glad of it, quite frankly. It shows prudence on your part. A driver without prudence is a fool."

"But we're losing."

Thomas shrugged. "I'll make it up for us this go-around, boyo." The pit crew backed off, and Thomas climbed into the DeManto. He winked at Morgan. "Next time I'll expect *you* to make it up for *me.*"

The next time Morgan did. It was like that first race had never happened. He took command of the DeManto prototype from the very first moments of his stint. Thomas and Morgan won that race, and the racing columns began to take note of the young American driver.

From that point on, Morgan took part in every manufacturers' race. He drove at Brands-Hatch, in England; the Monza, in Italy; the Sebring and Daytona Beach events in America; and the showcase 24 Heures du Mans, in France. The DeManto team placed well in every run. Professor DeManto threw a gala party at the ivy covered mansion to celebrate, and Morgan found himself the center of the racing media's attention. That same evening, Lee Thomas confided that his DeManto contract was up, and that for the upcoming season he had accepted a "ride"—financial backing, and a Formula One car—from another manufacturer. Morgan was summoned to Professor DeManto's study, where he found the tall, thin, white haired old man beautifully turned out in black tie, standing before a table on which rested the Championnat des Marques trophies the team had garnered. His gnarled hands hovered above the cups as if they were generating warmth. Morgan had seen the old man around the grounds, of course, but this was the first time he'd seen the Professor up close: his white curls, wide, patrician nose, and clear black eyes made him look like a perfectly preserved, or, perhaps, reincarnated, Roman emperor.

DeManto turned to Morgan and smiled. *"Grazie, Donaldo . . ."* The old man's hoarse, whispery Italian continued for a while, and then an assistant translated: "The *Professore* thanks you for bringing him these pretty things, and wishes to offer you his sponsorship for the upcoming Grand Prix season . . ."

Morgan was twenty-one years old, and a full-fledged Grand Prix driver.

That next season, out from under Thomas' protective, somewhat restraining wing, Morgan began to live it up. Thomas had rules about drinking and partying: for the forty-eight hours before a race he didn't touch a drop and got to bed early. Morgan had followed those rules out of deference to his boss when he'd been part of the Thomas circus, but now that he had a circus of his own, he did what he wanted and found that his natural ability allowed him to burn the candle at both ends and still win races.

As Morgan moved up in the Grand Prix standings the media was quick to adopt the handsome, chic, young American who was showing the Europeans how driving was done. Morgan was photogenic. He did a couple of cameos in James Bond type spy romps, and he was careful to see to it that the films showed him with the latest model DeManto sports car. The DeManto organization was pleased with the publicity and extended his contract. Soon offers for stateside television commercials began rolling in, and Morgan was forced to add a business manager to his circus.

Meanwhile, his relationship with Lee Thomas was changing. They were competitors and equals now, at least as far as Morgan was concerned; and maybe he was getting cocky, maybe he thought himself to be more than Lee's equal . . . In any event, at some race Thomas tore into him about his indulgent life-style, and Morgan told him where to get off. That pretty much ended their protege/mentor relationship, and their friendship. Morgan told himself that Thomas was jealous . . .

When he wasn't driving, Morgan was living in London, in a seven room, terraced flat near Regents Park. He was buying his clothes on Carnaby Street and King's Road, and going to a different "happening" every night. He experimented with grass, and acid, but the "head" thing wasn't his bag. He worried that drugs would dull his competitive edge. He stuck with champagne, and merely pretended to smoke grass when it was handed to him.

He often found himself still thinking about Ilsa, fantasizing about how she would throw herself at his feet now that he was a "somebody." But she was a somebody now, too: her modeling career had taken off; she was always popping up on magazine covers and in fashion layouts. Often he'd dream about her. Morgan was keeping his bed filled, but more out of habit and the need for a little physical relaxation than any heartfelt passion. It probably would have continued on like that if he hadn't gone to an album promotional party at Apple Recording Studios, where he saw Ilsa Wolff.

She was, of course, surrounded by a cluster of admirers. She was wearing dark, floral patterned stockings, black high heels, and a black velvet dress dusted with sequins. She was wearing her hair shorter, but otherwise she looked exactly as she had when Morgan had first seen her: astoundingly, impossibly beautiful.

Perhaps Ilsa felt his eyes upon her. She turned to him. She had a mesmerizing smile.

Morgan found himself moving across the room towards her, and then Ilsa was stepping into his arms. She moved close to kiss him, and Morgan felt an electric charge as his fingers brushed her hips canting forward beneath the black velvet. Her mouth was deliciously cool.

"Darling, how wonderful to see you again," she said in her languorous, German tinged English. "I've missed you so, and you've been so cruel not to call me . . ."

They left the party in order to find a quiet spot for a drink. It was almost eleven, and London shuts down early. Morgan had memberships in a couple of clubs where you could get drinks, drugs, boys, girls, or any combination thereof until the wee hours of the dawn, but the clubs were raucous, see-and-be-seen places.

What he wanted was a spot where they could be quietly, anonymously alone. He didn't dare suggest she come back with him to his flat. With Ilsa he felt as tentative and awkward as a schoolboy nervously anticipating his first kiss. It was an awkwardness that was at once both exquisite and painful. It was love.

He slowly guided the white DeManto hardtop coupe he was driving that month around the theater districts of Piccadilly, Soho, and Covent Garden, eyes peeled for a place that might offer posttheater supper. He tried to concentrate on the road, and not bashing into a lamp post, but it wasn't easy. She was sitting just inches away; her perfume, a heady mix of violets and tea, filled the cockpit interior. When he reached for the gear stick his fingers kept brushing her knee. She laughed, playfully accusing him of touching her on purpose. He blushed (for what seemed the first time in a hundred years). She saw it (how she did, by the red light aura of the instrument panel, he'd never know), laughed again, placed her hand upon *his* knee, and that time he almost *did* run them off the road.

They decided upon a Convent Garden cafe that was just winding down for the evening. It had leather banquets, red and white checkered tablecloths, and framed, antique theatrical posters. The maitre d' was adamant that the kitchen was closed and there could be no more seatings, but Ilsa smiled at him, and the guy melted. And then they were at a corner table. Morgan got a sleepy waiter to bring them a bottle of Roederer, and leave them alone.

They talked their way through two hours and another bottle of champagne. Morgan told her all about himself, and she talked about her own past. She was the daughter of a financier, and had grown up in a world of finishing schools, servants, and holidays in the Black Forest.

"My brothers are brains, but I am not very smart. At least not the way you need to be in school. But that is all right. My parents are well satisfied by me." She paused. "My father breeds ponies, you see. It does not matter what they have inside." She tapped her chest. "It does not matter about their heart and soul. What matters is how they look. Well, it is my job to be daddy's beautiful girl." She grinned. "I am very good at my job."

The waiters had finished putting up the chairs on the tables all around them, and it was only a matter of moments before they would start wet mopping the floor.

Ilsa gestured towards their own yawning waiter a few paces away. "We should go."

Morgan said, "I don't want to say goodnight."

"This is foolish, Donald. We should go to your flat." She looked innocently inquisitive. "I think that you have been waiting for me a very long time."

A half hour later their clothes were scattered on the floor of Morgan's candlelit bedroom, and they were rolling and tumbling on his wide, four poster bed. All the way home Morgan had worried that he had invested too much emotional importance in all this; that he wouldn't be able to get it up or that he would come too fast. They were needless, foolish worries. Just the touch and taste of her had him hard as a rock, and when he was inside her he knew that he could stay there forever, because there wasn't a molecule of his body that wanted this bliss to end.

Ilsa was sweating and squealing and moaning when they fell *off* the damned bed. The two of them cried out in shock, and then began to laugh hysterically. It occurred to Morgan that this was the first time he'd laughed during sex. God, he'd been missing a lot by not being with his love . . .

Ilsa was trying to clamber up off the floor but Morgan pulled her down, slid inside her again, and then climbed to his feet with their bodies locked together. Ilsa arched her back, her arms around his neck, and her thighs around his waist. She pumped against him as he danced with her around the room. As his own orgasm began bubbling at the base of his spine he managed with the last bit of strength in his rubbery legs to hurl them back on the bed.

The next thing he knew she was looking down at him in concern. Her cropped hair hung in damp ringlets of spun gold, and her almond eyes were wide. "Do you always pass out?"

"First time for everything."

Ilsa slumped beside him on her back, languidly stretching and arching. "I have never been so well fucked in my life," she said lazily. Her tongue darted into Morgan's ear. "First time for everything, hmm?"

Morgan kissed her. "I love you."

"Do you really? And as much as I think?" She sounded truly awed.

"Now and always," he said, and rolled on top of her.

"What is this now?" Her fingers were busy between his legs. *"Ach!* Again? So soon?

"Now that I've got you I may not let you go," Morgan warned, descending upon her.

"We will see who holds who captive," Ilsa warned, smiling her Mona Lisa smile as her body entwined with his upon the rumpled sheets.

Later, while she was in the bathroom, Morgan began to scoop up their things scattered across the bedroom floor. When he picked up Ilsa's purse it came open, and out fell a number of small, folded, paper packets. He opened one, it was full of fine white powder with a pretty sheen to it.

He heard the bathroom door open, and Ilsa come back into the room. "What are these?" Morgan asked.

"Mine," Ilsa said fiercely, her hand outstretched, palm up.

"Hey, what's the big deal." He gave her back her little packets. She hurriedly tucked them into her purse.

While she was busy doing that Morgan put the packet he had palmed in between the pages of a book lying on the night table. The next day he asked a knowledgeable friend what the pretty white powder with the glossy sheen was. The friend dabbed a bit onto his pinkie and tasted it. He winked. "Heroin," he said.

So Morgan knew that Ilsa was snorting heroin from the beginning. He just didn't know enough about it to be alarmed, or maybe he just didn't *want* to know enough about it. Maybe he was afraid that if he pushed Ilsa too hard he'd lose her. Even after they were married he never really felt like she belonged to him. Their first year of married life began well. Morgan was winning races, and Ilsa was by his side. Then she received a spate of modeling assignments, and soon they hardly saw each other. Once they were separated for two months, and Morgan found himself missing her so much that it was affecting his performance on the track. Finally he couldn't bear it any longer. He turned an upcoming race over to a back-up driver and flew home to London, intending to surprise her.

He surprised her.

He found her all alone in the flat, stoned out of her mind on the hard stuff: one of his neckties was tightly knotted around her upper arm, and a syringe was hanging from its needle out of her bulging vein. She was lying curled up on the floor in a corner of the living room, surrounded by dozens of glossy studio photos of herself that had fallen from her black leather modeling portfolios.

"So young and pretty," Ilsa mumbled to him as her fingers gently caressed the images of herself in the photos. "Darling?" she asked Morgan, her voice hideously slurred. "Who is that pretty, young girl?"

Later, when she'd come down, she couldn't seem to explain her habit, or maybe Morgan was too busy crying to hear what she was trying to tell him. All she kept saying was, "It has nothing to do with you, darling. I love you so much. Never think that it has anything to do with you. . . ."

From then on things went steadily downhill. He exhausted himself trying to fulfill his responsibilities to DeManto and flying home to see her as often as he could. It didn't help. Her use of hard drugs increased. What was supposed to be their second anniversary celebration ended with both of them in tears as Ilsa admitted that she was no longer working. Her habit had ravaged her health and her looks, and with them had gone the modeling assignments. "You tell everyone that I am very busy working," she commanded him. "I am very serious, darling. I am very proud."

All he could see was the evil constellation of red sores crawling up her arms. "The tracks of my tears," he tried to joke, and bent his head to kiss them better, but Ilsa, grimacing, pulled away.

"Don't you pity me," she warned. "If you do I'll drive you away from me, and then *I* will pity *you*."

When he was with her she seemed rational. Yes, she knew how much he loved her, and yes, she would go somewhere to get help—but she would do it *next* week. Not today. Each time he returned to the Grand Prix circuit Morgan begged her to come with him.

"Darling," she shook her head. "The Grand Prix is yours. If I am not at the center of attention, I wither."

Maybe if he had stayed with her he could have helped her fight her addiction, but he *had* to drive, it was his job. . . .

His job. His driving luck had begun to unravel. He pinned some of the blame on a string of mechanical mishaps, but he knew that all the worrying about Ilsa had ruined his concentration, dulled his edge. These days he was drinking a little more, but he was handling it. Anyway, he needed some release. There were the pressures of driving, and at night, alone—he was always faithful to Ilsa—he agonized about where she was and what she was doing to herself. He couldn't call her; it enraged her to have him checking up. But if he didn't call, he was left with long, dark hours in which to imagine the worst, and then it would be time to drive again, and maybe he *was* drinking a little *too* much, but he could handle it.

He was in Sicily, for the Targa Florio cross-country race, that first time Ilsa overdosed. When the call came from London, he pulled his team out of competition. He knew DeManto would be furious, but the Targa Florio was far too treacherous a run to trust to apprentices.

He was back in London within a few hours and went directly from the airport to the hospital, where the doctors told him that they'd done all they could; now the fight belonged to his wife. Morgan sat by the bed, holding Ilsa's hand, willing her to live. When she opened her eyes he told her, "I said I wouldn't let you go."

Ilsa started crying then, promising to get clean, telling him that it wasn't too late for them to have a family. Morgan believed her: he *wanted* to believe her.

He wired the DeManto organization to request a six week leave of absence, which they seemed inordinately eager to grant. During that time he and Ilsa lived like an old retired couple. She went "cold turkey" from heroin, as he did from the booze. They went for walks each day in the park, and went to bed early. They didn't have sex. It seemed enough just to fall asleep in each other's arms. Ilsa got herself a job as a fashion photographer's assistant. Morgan decided that it was time for him to go back to his own work. He wired the DeManto organization, informing them that he was ready to rejoin his circus, but he received a reply asking him to come to the factory which he thought was odd. Nonetheless, he made arrangements to travel to Modena. He wanted Ilsa to come along with him, but she had her new job. Morgan said that he loved her very much.

Ilsa said, "But you also love your cars, darling." She laughed wistfully. "I will never get used to sharing the limelight."

The last thing Morgan noticed was that the sores on her arms had begun to fade.

In Modena one of Professor DeManto's assistants was waiting at the gate to escort Morgan to the ivy covered mansion, and then up to the same, somber, book-lined study where, two seasons ago, the Professor had offered him his ride.

The old man was seated in a high-backed leather armchair before a fire crackling in the hearth. Without looking at Morgan, he began to speak in Italian. He went on for what seemed to be minutes. When he was done, the assistant translated. "The *Professore,* he has known for some time about your marital problems. He has not communicated with you about them because he believes that what happens in a man's household," the translator paused, looking uncomfortable. "The *Professore* believes that is a man's own business. But your performance on the track, it has suffered, and that *is* the *Professore's* business. What is more, he is aware that you drink to excess. Not only does this cause your performance to suffer, but it also puts our expensive automobiles at risk. The *Professore,* he can afford to lose a car; he would not be a participant in racing if he could not, but he wishes for the odds to be in his favor as much as possible. Accordingly, he wishes to inform you that your contract with us has been terminated."

Morgan felt dizzy; felt as if he'd been locked into an ugly dream. *He was losing his ride. He would no longer be allowed to drive—*

He thought about Ilsa: she was going to blame herself for this. He could hear her crying about how sorry she was; about how she was no good for him . . . No! This couldn't happen! Not to him, and not to his *wife,* not now, when she was beginning to get better!

Morgan looked at a side table, on which were displayed the many cups he had won for DeManto. The old man saw him looking and seemed to wince. Professor DeManto said something else, which the assistant duly translated. "The *Professore*, he is grateful for all that you have done for DeManto, Signore Morgan. He wishes you to know that he lives for the day when he can repay the favor."

Morgan stared at the old man. *You two-faced sonofabitch,* is what he wanted to say, but he struggled to get control of his temper. "He can repay me now," Morgan said, forcing calmness into his voice. "By letting me drive for him again."

"Signore Morgan—" the assistant began.

"Listen to me!" Morgan pointed at the Professor. "Get *him* to listen to me." He was sounding desperate now, but he no longer cared. "The Professor needs me!" *And I need him,* Morgan added to himself.

"Donaldo." Professor DeManto had stood up, and now his dark, pain-wracked eyes were staring deeply into Morgan's own. "My *Inglese*, it is very little," he struggled. "This *decisione*, she . . . breaks my heart."

"Professor, with all due respect," Morgan began. "There are no more than thirty men in the world who can drive Grand Prix—"

"Donaldo," DeManto interrupted quietly, sorrowfully, finally. "There are now, I think, only twenty-nine."

It was not until Morgan had been ushered out of the old man's presence that the reality of what had just happened hit him, and his fury erupted. All during the flight home Morgan thought about what he should have said to that old bastard, DeManto. *Fuck him,* Morgan thought, seething inside. *Fuck that ignorant, old sonofabitch!* He hoped DeManto was satisfied with his table full of trophies, because without Don Morgan behind the wheel, DeManto's first places were going to be a thing of the past!

Morgan's anger cooled only when he began to ponder how to break the news to Ilsa. It wouldn't do to upset her, not when she was making such progress in defeating her drug addiction. Fortunately, they wouldn't have to worry about money. Most of what he'd made doing those commercial endorsements had been banked. Of course, the commercial endorsements were going to disappear once word got around that DeManto had fired him.

By the time the cab had dropped him at his flat Morgan's rage had crystallized into bitter indifference. He would be, as the French put it, *sans souci* . . . without care. He'd even come around to thinking that his being fired was a blessing in disguise. He'd been too long with DeManto. There were other car manufacturers; there were other rides. He'd get something, and if it turned out to be less financially advantageous than what he'd had, so what? He'd work his way back up to a championship, and then he'd once again be able to write his own ticket. Professor DeManto would beg him to come back, and then he could kick that old bastard in the teeth—just the way the Professor had kicked him.

The important thing was not to upset Ilsa.

The stereo was on, tuned to an FM rock station, when he let himself into the flat. He called out, but there was no answer. It occurred to him that she might be out working for that photographer, but then why would the stereo be on?

He went into the kitchen and the first thing he saw was the syringe, shattered into glistening shards, lying on the floor in a pool of clear liquid. Ilsa, wearing a chambray workshirt with fancy embroidering and a pair of faded, denim bell bottoms, was sitting on a chair, slumped over the kitchen table, her chin resting on her folded arms. She was expressionless, myopically gazing at the bottle cap, and matches, and open paper packets lying inches from her nose.

Too stoned to even know I'm here, Morgan thought. The frustration and rage—over the way DeManto had treated him, and over his disappointment in Ilsa—were boiling over in him. He screamed at her, but she was too stoned to hear him. He kicked the chair out from under her, lifted her up by the front of her workshirt, and shook her, and that's when he realized she was dead.

Somewhere, far out on the predawn, dark, cold waters of San Francisco Bay, a boat joined in woeful chorus with the braying fog horn. Nicole stirred in her sleep, and turned towards Morgan to nuzzle close. By the bedside lamp's soft light he studied her face, relaxed and open in sleep. He noticed crow's-feet around her eyes, and wondered her age. She wasn't as young as her terrific body made her seem.

Morgan kissed the crow's-feet, lightly, so as not to disturb her. He liked them fine. These days he favored things built to last.

Morgan opened his eyes. He looked at his watch. It was a little after six in the morning, and Nicole wasn't in bed with him. He saw light spilling from around the edge of the partly closed bedroom door, and could have sworn he heard the creak of a drawer being pushed shut.

"Nicole?" he called out sleepily.

"Yes! Yes, darling!"

It sounded to Morgan like she was calling out from the study. He wondered what she was doing in there, and thought about getting out of bed to investigate, but then she was back, crawling into bed beside him.

"I couldn't sleep, darling," she murmured, cuddling close. "I didn't want to disturb you . . ."

"It sounded like you were in my study." He was drifting off.

"Go to sleep, silly boy," she scolded lightly. And he did.

4

MORGAN WOKE UP at eight. Nicole wasn't in bed with him. He called out, but got no answer. Somehow he wasn't surprised.

He got out of bed, wrapped a robe around himself, and explored the apartment. Nicole had totally cleaned up after herself. The ashtrays had been emptied. The two wine glasses had been washed. The empty wine bottle was in the trash.

She hadn't left a note. Hell, she hadn't even left fingerprints. Nicole Houel was one weird woman.

He thought about how he was sure that she'd been rummaging through his desk drawers in his study last night, and went in to take a look around. The study was more cluttered than the rest of the apartment. There was a long leather couch, and the pugnacious rolltop desk, both of which Morgan had found lying neglected in the backroom of an antique shop in Jackson Square. There were Persian rugs, vibrant as flowers in bloom, and floor-to-ceiling shelves crammed with books, and stereo and television components.

Everything looked in its place, but then Morgan wasn't the sort of neatness freak who'd notice if some papers had been moved around. He went to his desk and opened the top drawer, hearing the same creak that he'd heard last night. He kept nothing but pencils, pens, and that sort of thing in this drawer, and Nicole hadn't stolen any of his paper clips as far as he could tell.

If Nicole had been in here, Morgan thought, the question was, what the hell was she looking for?

As he wandered out of the study he noticed himself in a mirror: a tall guy with dark hair cut short and salted with gray, wearing nothing but a red cotton terrycloth robe and perplexed expression.

Morgan laughed out loud and went into the kitchen to start the coffee brewing. He put the entire Nicole Houel mystery out of his mind as he showered and shaved. She was a journalist, after all, and she'd told him that she was writing a story about Niles Kingman. Maybe she'd had doubts about Morgan's claim that he wasn't all that close to Niles, and had been prowling around in his study to find evidence to the contrary?

No matter. Morgan had bigger fish to fry: like what he was going to do about the fact that someone had leaked his closely guarded expansion plans to Kingman?

He brooded about the leak in his organization as he ate breakfast, and then he remembered last night's broadcast waiting for him on the VCR. He took his coffee into the study, switched on the tube, and re-wound the tape. He was feeling a little nervous. He'd been in *People*, and *Time;* and there'd been lots of profiles in the automotive magazines, but this was his debut on prime time, network television news.

Morgan fast-forwarded through the show's opening credits, to the beginning of his segment. He watched the filmed history of his racing career. At least he guessed it was his career: he didn't feel like he even knew that scrawny kid in goggles and helmet grinning back at him from inside the Sony.

The racing footage segued into clips from his numerous television commercials, and then there was suddenly a clip of Ilsa when she was healthy and happy and beautiful, hugging him after he'd won some race. In the background was a cheering crowd in a grandstand. Close by, anonymous hands triumphantly held aloft a silver cup and foaming bottles of Perrier-Jouët. Morgan, still in his driving gear, and Ilsa, a blonde goddess in slinky black, embraced before the blood red DeManto Formula One, its lithe fenders glistening with spilled champagne.

Morgan quickly blanked it from his mind and his heart, and zapped away the pretty picture memories with the VCR's remote control.

He realized that he hadn't been paying attention to the voiceover. He rewound the tape to listen to what the show's host, an avuncular, veteran newsman, had to say:

". . . You may remember Don 'Donnie' Morgan from the sixties. He was that dark-haired, Steve McQueen lookalike, the one who made a lucrative career out of hawking everything from motor oil to razor blades when he wasn't breaking speed records on the Grand Prix racing circuit.

"Then came tragedy: Morgan's wife, sixties supermodel, Ilsa Wolff, shown here congratulating her husband after a successful race, died of a drug overdose, and Morgan's racing career began to run out of gas.

"The DeManto organization fired him, and Morgan had a brief, unsuccessful career as a network sports commentator on the racing scene."

Morgan stared dully at footage showing the DeManto complex in Modena; and himself, in an ill-fitting, network blazer, shoving a microphone at a disinterested driver.

"It was the Fleet Street newspapers that broke the story of Morgan's bout with the bottle. He denied that he was an alcoholic, and threatened to sue for libel, but the threat of litigation faded away, as did Don Morgan."

They showed those ancient, ugly, banner headlines run by the London rags, along with those infamous photos taken of him with a telescopic lens while he was trying to dry out in that supposedly exclusive, supposedly *discreet* Swiss sanitarium he'd checked himself into.

"Morgan's second chance came when his old mentor,

51

Lee Thomas, offered Morgan a spot on his BXI Grand Prix racing team—"

Morgan watched himself and a smiling Lee Thomas putting their arms around each other's shoulders in front of reporters at a news conference. Morgan watched and listened, dreading what was coming next.

"This was Morgan's second chance, but it, too, ended in tragedy: at the 24 hour endurance event at Le Mans. Morgan was Lee Thomas' relief driver. Thomas, and then Morgan, had driven brilliantly during their stints behind the wheel in this grueling race, but then, during his second stint, Lee Thomas lost control of the team's BXI racer."

Morgan tried, but could not avert his eyes as the television screen was filled with the image of the pine green, BXI Formula One emerging from beneath the Le Mans Dunlop Bridge, suddenly skidding, and then bursting into flame as it cartwheeled off the track.

"Immediately after the accident, rumors swirled that Don Morgan was somehow to blame for Lee Thomas' crash. But then the chief mechanic of the BXI team pit crew issued a statement blaming brake failure for the accident.

"With Morgan's name and reputation cleared, offers to drive—'rides' in track parlance—poured in, but Morgan, distraught over Lee Thomas' death, accepted none of them. For the second time in his life, Morgan seemed to disappear off the face of the earth.

"You may have wondered, whatever happened to Donnie Morgan?"

The old racing history and commercial clips segued to a montage of the parking lots on Rodeo Drive, the camera lovingly caressing the exoticar fleets of Ferraris and Porsches. The host's voiceover continued:

". . . This is what happened to Donnie Morgan. In the world of glitter, Donnie Morgan is a 'candy man'; a purveyor of seductive and illicit things to those who can pay. But instead of drugs, Morgan deals cars, the wildest, most exotic machines the automotive wizards of

Europe have to offer. Deemed too potent for the U.S. market by their manufacturers, these gray market dream machines are what the status-conscious—with hundreds of thousands of dollars burning holes in their pockets— naturally have to have.

"Here's 'Viewpoint' correspondent, Hank Conroy, with a profile of Donnie Morgan: 'Making a Fortune in the Fast Lane . . .'"

Morgan watched himself being interviewed; explaining how the automobile gray market worked: he crisscrossed Europe, purchasing the exoticars, and importing them to his Oakland test track facility DonSport, Ltd., where they were modified to meet the Environmental Protection Agency and Department of Transportation's standards. He grew uncomfortable, even a bit angry, when publicity stills of various actresses turned up in the segment, and the reporter linked them to him romantically. It was true that he'd had relationships with those women, but none of them had been especially serious . . . Anyway, even *People* had left that aspect of his life alone . . .

Next up was one of the editors from *Car* Magazine, a guy Morgan knew, who killed some airtime with psychobabble about why status symbol automobiles are so important in Hollywood.

Then they cut to a spokesman from the North American Alliance of Foreign Auto Dealers, who insisted that a weakening dollar had made gray market luxury automobiles an unwise investment. The *Car* magazine editor came back on to suggest that Morgan didn't sell investments, he sold exclusivity.

The segment ended with a chat between the anchorman and the correspondent. The host asked what the future held for Donnie Morgan.

Morgan expected the usual meaningless chitchat. He was not prepared for the correspondent's bombshell:

". . . Don Morgan has been secretly negotiating with a San Francisco–based investment banking firm to finance his bid to go nationwide with a chain of

DonSport, Ltd. boutiques, selling and supporting the most expensive gray market automobiles in the world, to the nation's most exclusive clientele."

Morgan sat in a state of shock as the host ended the segment with a rhetorical wrap up:

". . . Can Don Morgan do for the nation's yuppies what he's done for the Hollywood crowd? Those in the know think it's the ultimate finish line, one that Don Morgan is destined to cross . . .

"Next, Patty Slade uncovers the latest scandal rocking the European art community as museums and galleries suffer a rash of thefts. After this message, 'Viewpoint' will return, with 'Someone Is Stealing the Great Art-works of Europe.'"

Morgan shut off the VCR. He'd gotten over being shocked. Now he was angry and worried: Who the hell had leaked that information, and how would Joe Weiner, his contact at the investment firm of Weiner, Carlson & Boyd, react to the news?

Morgan flashed on how Niles Kingman had known about his expansion plans *yesterday afternoon.* This show hadn't been broadcast until *last night.* Whoever had leaked the information had talked to others besides the "Viewpoint" correspondent. Morgan had told only a few, highly trusted people at DonSport of his plans. He couldn't believe that any of those people would betray him. The leak had to have come from someone at Weiner, Carlson & Boyd.

Morgan thought about the call that had come in to his car phone answering machine last night, just about the time "Viewpoint" was being aired. He went to his desk and dug the apartment's answering machine out from beneath a drift of paperwork. The machine's red message indicator light was blinking.

Morgan played back his messages. There were a spate of congratulatory calls from the few close friends who knew his unlisted number, and, as expected, a very curt one from Joe Weiner: "Call my office, ASAP."

* * *

Morgan called Weiner, and arranged to see him in an hour. He called his own office and said he'd be in late. He dressed in dark blue, double-breasted, tropical weight wool, a white shirt, and a garnet tie. He checked the mirror. He looked great and felt awful. The tie was the color of spilled blood. How appropriate, Morgan thought. The blood would likely be his own. He had a sinking feeling in the pit of his stomach that his Harvé Benard clad hide was about to be nailed to the wall.

It was too late to extricate himself from the expansion venture. He'd already committed his own resources, putting all of his assets on the line to make the dream happen.

Currently, DonSport, Ltd. was extremely successful, but it was, well, limited; a definite, but circumscribed success. By going national, Morgan could tap into markets that were presently unavailable to him.

He could be at the top.

The best, at last.

It hadn't happened for him driving. Or maybe it was more that he hadn't let it happen. He'd had the potential to be a great champion, but he'd betrayed himself.

What the hell. Driving was in the past; his DonSport expansion plans were here and now—if Weiner didn't cut his financial legs out from under him.

All right, say the worst was going to happen, he hypothesized, that Weiner was going to pull his investment firm's money out of the deal, turning Morgan's ambitious dreams to ashes, and causing him to lose what he already had. Morgan had been penniless, down and dirty before, and had managed to get himself back on top.

He studied his mirror reflection: the graying hair, and the lines around his eyes. He'd been a hell of a lot younger last time he'd tumbled. He wasn't sure he had the strength to survive this time around if he found himself back at the bottom again.

"It's not fair," Morgan's reflection seemed to scowl.

He felt haunted by his past; doomed to repeat the bitter, frustrating cycle of brief success followed by devastating failure.

First time around, he had no one to blame but himself for having fucked himself over with booze, but this time he was being betrayed, by someone he trusted. Who was it? Which friend was his enemy?

Morgan turned away from the mirror, feeling sick and helpless. God, a drink would taste good . . .

Have one, the itty-bitty, frankfurter red, cartoon devil hopping up and down on his shoulder whispered in his ear. *Your financing looks blown. You're going to lose everything. You're dreams are shit. Have a drink. It'll calm you. Have a—*

"Fuck it—"

Morgan went into the kitchen and pulled out the fixings for a Bloody Mary. He mixed it just the way he liked it: double shot of vodka; chilled V-8 juice; splash of Tabasco and a dollop of Lea & Perrins; a sprinkling of celery seed and wedge of lemon.

It looked gorgeous and smelled ambrosial. He lifted the moisture beaded tumbler, carried it to the sink, and poured it down the drain, muttering obscene insults at the drink until it was gone. He rinsed the glass and put it in the dishwasher.

The little red devil had split. For now.

In the mornings he made Bloody Marys. At night it was usually a nice, big Wild Turkey on the rocks, with a splash of soda. He had the luckiest sink in town.

Weiner, Carlson & Boyd occupied an eagles' aerie a couple of floors beneath the pyramid shaped Transamerica building's pointy head. It had a reception area done up in corporate "Star Trek" mode: gleaming white walls, gray carpeting, black leather modular seating, and everything as quiet as a tomb but for the beehive whirr and muted clickety-clack of myriad, unseen computers.

The receptionist was seated behind a steel and white marble desk the size of an MGB. She was blonde, with pale blue eyes, and lashes the color of spider silk. Morgan identified himself and who he was here to see. The receptionist repeated that into a telephone. A few moments later a secretary appeared to lead Morgan around behind the snowy blonde and her snowy desk, through a steel door, and then past a maze of secretarial pools and busy corridors, to Weiner's office. The secretary knocked once on the door, and opened it for Morgan.

Weiner's office was appropriately plush and cavernous, but perversely old-fashioned, considering the place's high tech front, and its origins in the seventies as a Silicon Valley venture capital firm. The walls were walnut paneled. There was a mammoth expanse of burgundy carpeting in need of mowing, and matching floor-to-ceiling drapes framing a view of the BankAmerica Building and the cityscape beyond. An antique, Western Union banjo clock ticking like a metronome hung on the wall behind Weiner's desk. Off to one side, a trio of small, Morisot pastels of children at play occupied the paneled space between sconces with green glass shades.

Joe Weiner was at his desk, barely visible behind stacks of manila folders.

"Don, hello." He rose and came around to shake hands. His jacket was off, and his tie was loosened. He had black framed bifocals hanging around his neck by a thin, gold chain.

Weiner was short, but solidly built, and had thick, wiry, dun colored hair brushed straight up. In happier, more flippant times Morgan had thought he kind of looked like a late-middle-aged Gumby. Today Morgan thought Weiner looked like doom.

"You want anything?" Weiner asked. "Coffee, anything?"

"Coffee," Morgan said.

Weiner nodded to the secretary in the doorway and she went away. Weiner led Morgan to a couple of tufted leather chairs in a corner of the room.

"I take it you wanted to see me because you caught last night's 'Viewpoint'?" Morgan asked once they were settled.

Weiner looked uncomfortable. "I did see it, and it's causing me a damned headache."

Weiner's phone warbled. He excused himself and went to answer it. Morgan used the time to formulate a strategy against what he knew was coming.

A DonSport client, a young software wizard who had sold his company for ten million and wanted to put some pocket change into a Maserati, had introduced Morgan to Weiner. With the slow-up in the computer industry, Weiner's venture capital firm had been looking to diversify. Morgan's expansion plans had initially interested them, but they'd cautioned Morgan that their firm had always kept a low public profile. The negotiations had to remain secret.

"I don't want any calls while I'm in this meeting," Weiner told whomever was at the other end of the line. He hung up and returned to the armchair. "Sorry about that." The secretary came in with a china coffee service on a silver tray. She poured them both cups from the Wedgewood pot. Morgan added a drop of cream to his, took a sip, and waited as Weiner dismissed the secretary. When she was gone, shutting the door behind her, Morgan said, "I think the leak about my expansion plans came from your office, Joe . . ."

"No way!" Weiner said. He looked offended. "We've spent almost two decades in the computer industry, which is probably the most secretive, leak-sensitive business in the world, and we've always maintained a spotless security record. Nobody in this office talked to 'Viewpoint.'"

"Okay," Morgan said. If you say so, he thought. He considered telling Weiner about his exchange with Niles Kingman, and that the cat had been let out of the bag before last night's airing of "Viewpoint," but decided against it. Weiner was already riled up. There was no sense in antagonizing a man from whom you wished to borrow twelve million dollars.

"What's happened is over and done with," Morgan said. "What are the ramifications?"

Weiner emptied a packet of Sweet and Low into his coffee, and gave it a desultory stir. "NAAFAD lawyers were on the horn to us first thing this morning, threatening litigation." He shrugged. "My firm has got to back off."

Don't freak, Morgan told himself. You suspected this was coming, so deal with it. NAAFAD was the North American Alliance of Foreign Auto Dealers. They'd considered Morgan and DonSport to be a potential threat from its beginning, but really began to hate his guts when the publicity he received began to rub off on lesser known gray market dealers.

"Joe, we've run countless spreadsheets on my proposal. You know that the DonSport expansion prospectus is rock solid."

"That is not the issue," Weiner began.

"And you know that the time is right to break the authorized dealers' stranglehold on the high-end, import market," Morgan argued. "NAAFAD's legal threats are all bluff. The DonSport boutiques will sell only gray market cars. The authorized dealers can't sue us for selling what they don't carry. And the various car manufacturers will back us up. There's been no love lost between them and NAAFAD since Adler Motors was sued by its independent dealer network to prevent the Stuttgart based company from opening direct factory-to-consumer sales centers."

"It's not the litigation that scares us, it's the attendant publicity," Weiner explained. "We're still doing a lot of business in Silicon Valley. We need to maintain a low profile. If we get involved in litigation, we'll make the newspapers. If the media starts digging at us, they might uncover some of our computer and software projects, all of which are at highly sensitive levels of development."

"Joe—"

"Morgan, let go of it for a while," Weiner advised. "Lay low."

"You know I can't," Morgan said. "I'm already in too deep. I've put up everything to borrow what I needed to lock in my options on real estate all across the country."

"For the dealerships . . ." Weiner nodded, and then sighed. "You know, at the time, I thought you were being hasty . . ."

"Thanks for the benefit of your hindsight," Morgan said wryly. "Lock the barn door on your way out, would you? I'm busy chasing after a missing horse."

"You can survive this," Weiner encouraged. "DonSport is doing very well. Arrange with your creditors to just pay interest, and let the principal ride. Hell, they let all of Latin America do it," he chuckled. "Why not DonSport? Like I said, just lay back a while, Morgan. Until all this publicity blows over. Then, maybe, we can get back on track—"

"*Maybe*, Joe?" Morgan frowned. "After everything, all you can give me is a *maybe?*"

"That's all," Weiner nodded. "That's all my partners will allow me to give. I need time if you want me to mend this agreement. Be reasonable. You can afford to give me that time. You're a millionaire several times over. You don't need the money—"

Morgan sipped at his coffee, but it had gone cold. He thought about telling Weiner about his personal reasons for wanting this expansion, but it made no sense to demean himself that way, especially since baring his personal demons to the man wouldn't make the slightest difference. This entire exchange had begun to remind him of the one he'd had years ago, with Professor DeManto, when he'd been told that he'd been fired. The Professor had made up his mind before Morgan had taken one step into the old man's study.

The actual meeting between the two had been a mere formality. So was this meeting: Weiner had made up his mind last night, while watching "Viewpoint." Right now, he was just showing Morgan a courtesy by pretending to discuss the situation.

"You realize that your firm is going to lose a lot of money by not backing me?" Morgan warned.

Weiner said, "I know."

Not much room for negotiation there, Morgan thought. He stood up. So did Weiner, who seemed indecently eager to walk him to the door.

"Keep one thing in mind," Weiner advised. "Whoever leaked this information wanted very badly to hurt you. If it's someone in your organization—which it has to be—someone you think is a friend . . ."

Morgan did not want to hear it. Weiner didn't care.

"—Morgan, with friends like that, who needs enemies?"

5

It was noon by the time Morgan made it back to his apartment to exchange the blue suit for a pair of jeans and a sweater. He got the attaché case full of cash out of the wall safe, and then drove over to the bank. Fifteen minutes, and assorted counts and filled-out government forms later, Morgan was on his way to DonSport.

Driving across the Oakland Bay Bridge and getting stuck in traffic southbound on the Nimitz Freeway gave him plenty of time to brood over which of his most trusted friends or associates was stabbing him in the back. For now, he was prepared to accept Weiner's assertion that the leak had come from DonSport. Weiner, Carlson & Boyd did have a spotless record when it came to discretion about their clients. It was simply more likely that the leak had come from one of his own people, which made the betrayal doubly bitter: the people who knew of his talks with Weiner had all been with DonSport for years.

Except for one person. Could Sonny Thomas have betrayed him? The motive was there, *if* Sonny had somehow managed to uncover the truth that Morgan had so carefully buried.

He passed the Oakland Coliseum, and moved to the right for his upcoming exit. He left the freeway, and five minutes later was nodding to the security guards on duty at DonSport's entrance gate.

"*Club Med for cars . . .*" one of the enthusiast magazines had called the place. Morgan was proud of the setup. The garage complex was equipped with state-of-the-art automotive diagnostic and repair equipment. His parts inventory was one of the most extensive in the country, and he had the contacts in America and abroad to get a part he didn't have—even a vintage part—air freighted.

Morgan drove past central parking, and the office and gym, towards the test track, DonSport's jewel in the crown. It was a 2.73 mile circuit of dips, rises, curves, and swerves; there were sections of dirt, gravel, and concrete, as well as asphalt; there was even a section with built-in sprinklers to allow his people to test various car and tire combinations for skidding and hydroplaning. The only driving conditions Morgan's test track couldn't duplicate were ice and snow, but most of the pretty toys DonSport sold—the German cars excluded—weren't meant to be taken on skiing trips.

Morgan pulled up alongside the track's pitstop area. Marty Robbins, resplendent in greasy mechanic's overalls and an LA Angels baseball cap, was at a table fiddling with a radar gun. As soon as Morgan switched off the BMW's engine he heard the faraway bee buzz. By the time he was out of his car and at trackside, the bee buzz had grown to a terrier's snarl, and then a lion's roar—

Robbins aimed his radar gun as the coal-black flash that was a DeManto 200 GTS zoomed by. The roar abruptly dropped off into a keening whine.

"Sexiest sound in the world," Morgan said.

Marty Robbins nodded as he put down the gun and made a note on the clipboard on the table. "The sound of a twelve cylinder engine. To know it is to love it."

Robbins was built wider than he was tall. He was pure toad-ugly. His nose was flattened, he had a glass eye, and lots of scar tissue, all the result of an episode when Robbins had pushed too hard, slamming a car into a retaining wall, and his head through the windshield.

Robbins' office and administrative staff were situated in the garage and parts complex. He was listed on the company's letterhead as "Vice-President and Executive Director of Diagnostics, Research, Development." In other words, he kept the status quo when Morgan was away, and was the head honcho grease monkey. Morgan had tried for years to get Robbins out of smudged overalls and into a suit. He'd succeeded once, but pretty soon Robbins' suit was smudged, and there were screwdrivers poking up out of his suit jacket's breast pocket, where the hanky was supposed to go. So Morgan gave up; he let Robbins be Robbins. Anyway, Robbins in a suit still looked like a toad; just one stuffed into Ken doll clothes.

Morgan gestured at the radar gun. "How fast?"

Robbins shook his head. "It would only break your heart to know." He grinned. "On second thought, 155."

"Dammit, Marty, that car is sold! I'd like to deliver it with its engine intact. Black flag it next time around."

"Just a few more laps," Robbins said. "I fitted her with some experimental rubber."

"The DonSport signature tires we've been working on with the Merite people?"

Robbins nodded. "We came up with a new compound. I want to see the wear patterns."

"Just don't blow that engine."

"Don't worry," Robbins said. He tapped at the clipboard with a blunt, grease-rimmed finger nail. "This car is checking out to be outstanding. Tracking and steering feel are exceptional for a DeManto." He looked hard at Morgan. "What I'd like to know is what's put the burr in your blanket today?"

Morgan turned away. "I'm sorry. Some shitty news. I'll fill you in later."

The bee buzz was back, quickly ascending to its roar,

and then dropping to its shrill, fading whine as the black blur sped past, the wind flapping both men's clothes.

"Is that Sonny?" Morgan asked.

Robbins laughed. "None other. Sonny is the only hot shoe we've got who will drive balls-out, which is what I needed on this go around. There's nothing that kid won't try."

Including selling me out? Morgan wondered. "Send Sonny to see me as soon as you two are done pounding that GTS into the ground."

"Your office?" Robbins asked.

"My office," Morgan said. He turned to go, then stopped. "Tell Sonny, I mean right away!"

"What you oughtta do is go exhaust yourself in the gym. You're getting like you-know-how-you-get."

For a split second Morgan felt like taking a swing at Robbins, but then he realized the only person he wanted to punch was himself. "Marty. I just came from Weiner's office. We lost our financing."

Robbins nodded and went back to his clipboard notes.

"You don't seem very surprised," Morgan said warily.

"What?" Robbins stared at him. "What the fuck do you mean by *that?*"

"I mean that it looks like somebody *here* leaked that information—"

"You want to get that tone out of your voice," Robbins said, "Or you want me to resign. Pick one."

"All I want," he began, struggling to keep his voice even, "is for you to explain why it comes as no surprise to you that we've just been knocked flat on our ass?"

"I saw that 'Viewpoint' thing," Robbins explained. "I heard them announce our plans to the fucking world. It's no surprise that a hinky guy like Weiner would chicken out after that."

"Yeah, I guess so." Morgan watched the black GTS roar by a third time. "Yeah, sure. That makes sense."

The car receded, then vanished around a curve. Morgan wished he could do the same. He felt like shit for suspecting his old friend. "I'm sorry, Marty."

"Shut up, boss." Robbins winked at him. "Does all this have to do with why you want to talk to Sonny?"

"I intend to talk to everyone who knew about the plans." Morgan said. "You and Sonny are pretty tight. I figure the two of you were in some bar seeing who could down the most boilermakers, and you got tanked and let it slip; am I right?"

"No, you're not right, dammit. I never told Sonny."

Morgan forced a sheepish smile. "Okay. So now I'm real sorry."

Robbins turned red. "Shit, I just remembered. I *did* tell Arthur."

"That's just great . . ." Morgan glared. "So now I'm *not* so sorry."

"I guess I made a mistake, Morgan." Robbins looked like he was in real pain. "It's just that . . . Well, you know how badly Arthur Neal and I have been getting along. It cost you so much to lure Neal away from Detroit to come work here . . . I knew that the friction between us was bothering you, so I figured that by telling him it would bring us closer together. See what I'm getting at?" he pleaded. "I get to be his buddy, and he quits complaining about me to you, like I *know* he's been doing—"

"Okay, Marty. I understand."

Robbins' shoulders were hunched in anguish. "All along I've been trying not to rock the boat, and there I went and damn well tipped it over!"

"Don't sweat it," Morgan said. "It was an error in judgment, that's all. We're not capsized, we're just ankle-deep in water. Anyway, we don't *know* that it was Arthur who gave out the information, and I'm glad you thought to tell me, because now I can add him to the list of people I need to talk to."

"But now *I'm* off it, right?"

"Right," Morgan said. A fucking white lie never hurt, and this was one he desperately wished were true.

Marty had been an essential player on the DonSport team right from its start, but it was no secret that lately he'd felt shunted aside by Arthur Neal. Morgan knew that Marty was a great guy, but an awful drunk; Marty was a brawler, a what-did-I-do-last-night? kind of drinker. Morgan could quite easily imagine Robbins having a few, working himself into a sodden, stuporous rage about Arthur Neal's rising star at DonSport, and making a telephone call to the "Viewpoint" correspondent. The punch line to this nasty joke was that Robbins, sobered up, would most likely have truly forgotten what he'd done. Or what he *might* have done . . .

"Morgan," Robbins was eyeing him carefully. "I know you're pissed off, but if I were you, I'd want somebody to remind me that this blow-out with Weiner is just like losing a race. It happens. No point kicking yourself in the ass. Just try to do better next time."

"It's a little different, Marty," Morgan said slowly, working it out in his own mind as he explained it to Robbins. "This is like losing a race because somebody in the pit crew fucked up on purpose."

"I hear you . . . But at least now you know that you don't have to worry about Sonny or me being the one?"

"I'll talk to you about it later, Marty."

"Just don't worry so much. We'll get the money somewhere else," Robbins was cheerleading. "There's no hurry. You know, except for that last bit where that reporter ate our lunch for us, I liked the broadcast. I thought it made us look real good."

"'And it's better to look good than to feel good?'" Morgan chuckled. "I'll see you later."

He got into the BMW and drove back to the office/gym complex. He entered the single story building through the reception area furnished with Recaro chairs, and decorated with the original Leroy Neiman paintings of DonSport locales commissioned by *Playboy* when it did its spread on the facility. Past reception, the front half of the complex was taken up by Morgan's private office, and the bookkeeping and import/export departments, arranged around word processing, records, and the telephone switchboard, like wagons around a campfire.

Beth, Morgan's secretary, looked up from her big desk, close to where the young woman operator sat playing her touchtone switchboard like a keyboard as she murmured into her headset.

"Nice of you to stop by," Beth said. "I was wondering if you still worked here."

Morgan grinned. When he'd first opened DonSport, he'd had this fantasy about hiring some sexy and savvy young lady; someone to play Effie Perrine to his Sam Spade. He was still looking for her when Beth came for an interview. She was savvy, but she was also a white haired black woman in her fifties, with a fishmonger's build and vocabulary. She favored a Margaret Thatcher style of dress: square cut wool suits and stubby heeled lace-up shoes. All in all, she was about as cuddly as a hatchet, but Morgan had hired her on the spot, on impulse, and it had proved to be the soundest business decision he'd ever made.

"What's doing?" Morgan asked.

"What *isn't doing* is the question," Beth muttered. "First of all you've got about eighty phone messages on your desk. Next, the customs broker called to say the six Audens we're waiting on are jammed up in a wildcat work stoppage in Hamburg. The computers are down in inventory supply, and some lawyer from NAAFAD has been phoning all morning demanding to speak to you and threatening to sue."

"Fuck NAAFAD."

"Too much work for one girl. I'll have to bring in some temps."

"I'll be in my office."

"What happened at Weiner, Carlson and Boyd?"

"You may officially remove them from the Rolodex."

"Chickenshits." Beth frowned. "So, what are we going to do now?"

"If I knew that, I'd be doing it," Morgan grumbled. "Not moping around here—"

Beth held up her hands in surrender. "Just a few things, darling. The 'Hyde and Seeker' television series called. They want to borrow a Mercedes 560 SEC convertible."

"Do we have one?" Morgan asked.

"One fresh out of the hands of Marty's elves."

"Lend it," Morgan said. "That show's hot. Orders jumped the last time they featured one of our cars. Just make sure we've got a copy of the production's insurance binder on the vehicle made out in our name, and that they've got a copy of our revised logo for their closing credits."

"They also wanted to know if you'd consider making a cameo appearance on the show."

"Get out of town," Morgan chuckled.

Beth giggled. "On the level, darling. You're a hot property since 'Viewpoint.'"

"Tell them I'm flattered, and thank them for asking, but no way. I've been that route, and it holds no further allure. What else?"

"Arthur Neal wants to see you."

Morgan shook his head. "Stall him."

"He's being rather insistent."

"He's always insistent." And I'm starting to regret the fact that I hired him, Morgan thought. "Do you know what he wants?"

"I think he's got a stick up his ass about Marty . . . for a change." Beth added.

"I'll see him later. Right now the only person I want to see is Sonny."

Morgan went into his office, settled into his own, custom-contoured, leather Recaro chair, and fidgeted at his desk, shuffling through his phone messages like they were a deck of cards. He decided that he'd been right the first time: they could all wait, to put it kindly, until hell froze over.

He was going to follow Weiner's advice and arrange with his creditors to pay only the interest on his loan. Morgan knew that they'd go for it, and while he would still be in a financially terrible position, it was, contrary to popular belief, often better to be in the frying pan as opposed to the fire.

Yes, he would make the call, and get that particular ball rolling: soon.

Right now, all he could think—make that brood—about, was who had stabbed him in the back, and when were they planning to plant the next blade?

Some purchase orders were crying out for attention at the top of his in box. Morgan grabbed one, scanned it, and picked up a pencil in order to initial it. The point of the pencil broke. Morgan snapped the pencil in two. Shards of wood flew up; they harmlessly bounced off his cheek. He swore and threw the bits of pencil across the room.

His scalp felt too tight for his skull. His skin itched. The last time he'd felt this bad had been years ago, one dark morning around four, when a real horror show of a craving for booze had converged on him like a swiftly moving storm front. He'd called somebody from AA, and they'd talked him down.

But today's evil eye had nothing to do with drink. Morgan remembered how it was when he was just a kid, starting out in stockcar racing. Morgan would work his way into the lead, but some asshole with a faster car would creep up on his tail, to give Morgan a bump on the rear. Morgan remembered how he would have his old Galaxie going flat-out, pedal to the metal, but that asshole in his monster Buick, or Pontiac, or Olds, would be stroking it, just laying back, enjoying being the cat to Morgan's mouse, and bump-bump-bumping his rear, until the moment came to pounce—

Morgan shook himself out of it. *Chrrrist . . .*

The term was *brain fade*, a bit of jargon cloned off

"brake fade." *Brain fade* referred to a driver's often lethal lapse of intelligence at a crucial moment. It meant midjudgment, confusion, computer overload; ordinary, garden variety stupidity. It meant the driver was faced with a crisis and didn't know what to do.

Morgan had brain fade. He was faced with a crisis, and he didn't know what to do. Sure, he could begin measures to get himself out of the money pit into which he'd been pushed, but no matter which way he jumped, no matter what his strategy, whoever it was on his tail had the position and power to counter it. Unless—until —Morgan found out who that person was.

He realized that his jaw ached. No wonder: he'd been gritting his teeth since the fiasco in Weiner's office. He had about eighty zillion watts of electricity zinging up and down his spine. Forget a masseuse. It'd take a jackhammer to get the kinks out.

He flashed on Marty's advice to work it all out in the gym. It made more sense than sitting here, uselessly vibrating with nervous frustration. It made more sense than courting an ulcer or a heart attack.

He buzzed Beth. "If anything exciting happens I'll be in the gym."

"You want to build up your muscles, try lifting your in box—"

"It'll all wait. Whatever it all is."

"Then have a nice time beating up your barbells."

He went into his private bath with its whirlpool and sauna, and used his key to unlock the connecting door that was his personal entrance into the gym that occupied the entire rear half of the building. In addition to Nautilus, free weight, and aerobic exercise equipment, there were locker rooms, showers, saunas, and whirlpools, all of which were open to employees, at lunchtime, on weekends, and before and after business hours.

Right now Morgan had the place to himself. He changed into sweats, put a Stanley Turrentine tape on the stereo system, and spent fifteen minutes stretching on the mats before tackling the twelve exercise Nautilus circuit. He took his time, blanking out his mind, concentrating on doing all of the exercises correctly, even the ones on the boring, lower body machines. Pretty soon he had worked up a sweat and was feeling a little looser; physically, if not mentally.

He was on the rotary torso machine when he heard the main door to the gym open and someone come in. He looked around, and was faced with what at first glance resembled a spaceman: a figure in a formless, dun colored jumpsuit; gloves, helmet, eyeport shield, nose shroud, and breathing filter.

"Very funny," Morgan said.

"You said as soon as possible," came a muffled voice from inside all that racing drag. "I drove the GTS straight over."

"You mean there still *is* a GTS?" Morgan scowled. He went over to the free weights area and began to set up a bench. "It's not all in a smouldering little pile alongside the track?"

"Except for a sore stickshift that big fellow is as good as ever," Sonny said. "Actually better than ever, now that I popped his cherry."

"Boys don't have cherries," Morgan said.

"Couldn't prove it by me." Sonny began to shed driving gear. "But I'm not one to quibble over produce. How's 'peel his banana?'"

Morgan laughed. He watched as off came Sonny's driving gloves and shoes, helmet, neck sock, and ski-mask-like flame retardant head covering.

God, she is beautiful, Morgan thought.

She was Morgan's height; a long, lean, brown eyed brunette with shoulder-length hair just now twisted up into a lopsided topknot. She was sheened with sweat, wearing only a skimpy pair of damp, baggy, white cotton running shorts, and a damp white T-shirt cut short to expose her midriff. The T-shirt hid little. Her nipples looked like BBs upholstered in white cotton.

Morgan felt himself responding to her, but his totally normal physical reaction made him feel funny; maybe even a little queasy, like when a guy catches himself ogling his sister . . . *That is Lee Thomas' daughter,* Morgan sternly reminded himself. There was a truckload of trouble from the past that separated them. It was Lee Thomas' ghost that reminded him to keep Sonny at arm's length.

Sonny finally kicked her feet free of the stiff, baggy fire suit. Morgan felt like he'd just watched a glistening butterfly wiggle free of a drab, brown cocoon.

"Mind if I work out with you?" Sonny asked.

Morgan nodded. "We can spot each other on the free weights."

He lifted 135 for his warm-up set. He racked the bar and loaded it with the appropriate plates and collars. Then he settled down on his back on the bench and got comfortable.

Sonny came over to spot him. She stood just behind and above Morgan, who was lying on the bench. Her legs were spread apart to brace herself in case she had to lift the weight off of him.

Her crotch was about a foot above his face. She smelled like a healthy young woman who had worked herself into a lather, but also, distractingly, of violets and tea. Morgan recognized the scent as the one Ilsa had favored. The coincidence gave him chills. He found it endearing that Sonny, his ace, hot-foot test driver, might feel the need to assert her femininity by dabbing herself with perfume before donning her macho racing gear.

As Morgan gazed up, a bead of moisture, lazily gliding from beneath Sonny's loose, high cut shorts, trailed the rounded curve of her inner thigh, before plunking onto Morgan's forehead. "You're dripping on me."

"I've heard that before," Sonny said, looking down at him. "Lift."

73

Morgan took the bar cleanly off the rack and cranked out a crisp series of twelve. "Your turn." He got off the bench. "What weight?" He prepared to remove the 45 pound plates from the bar.

"This will be fine."

"Sonny, 135 is too heavy for you," Morgan warned. "Just because I did it—"

"Leave it," she stubbornly insisted. "I can lift it, Morgan." She settled into position on the bench. Her long, tan thighs were taut as she straddled the bench, her nut brown toes flexing at the carpet, her round butt and the small of her back pressed against the padding.

Morgan went around behind the bench, dead certain he was going to have to save her when the 135 pounds went crashing down towards her chest. Sonny gripped the bar, took a deep breath, and let out a karate yell as she took the bar cleanly off the rack and held it motionless above her for a moment before letting it slowly sink to her chest. She took another deep breath and let it out as she tried to raise the barbell: she wrestled it a few inches higher, then got stalled. Morgan reached down to take it off of her.

"Stop, dammit!" She harshly grunted. "I've got it!"

Morgan stepped back. "Okay," he said flatly, surprised and a little put off by the ferocity of her tone. He watched her struggle with the bar, not quite able to beat it, but not yet surrendering. Her eyes were closed, and her face was flushed.

She's having sex with the damn thing, Morgan thought.

Her lips parted as she puffed with effort. Her breasts were splayed, the aureoles dark rings beneath stretched white cotton as her arms flexed and corded against the weight. With a long, groaning exhalation, she shoved the barbell towards the ceiling.

"That's outstanding!" Morgan said as her arms straightened.

"That's it," she moaned. Morgan took hold of the

bar, guiding it as she set it back into the rack. Sonny went limp, melting onto the bench.

"Told you I could do it," she gasped, trying to catch her breath.

"Sorry about trying to take it from you too soon. I really didn't think you could."

"I know, Morgan," Sonny said as she swung off the bench and faced him. "You *always* underestimate me."

"I'll remember that," Morgan said.

"Please try to do so," She quickly replied, very serious now.

Morgan let her have the last word. He always let Sonny's brattiness slide by, recognizing it for what it was: a feminine version of typical macho track bravado. Sure, she came on too strong and too pushy, but she was a hot foot, a pro driver. Her cocksure arrogance served as an emotional buffer against stress, as it served most race drivers, and for all Morgan knew, as it served test pilots, and deep sea divers, and anyone else who routinely did horrifically dangerous things. Morgan had been there; he remembered how it was.

He also knew some drivers who were quiet and unassuming, but they were older, more mature; they could let their brilliant careers do the talking.

Sonny had it within her to be that great, or as great as any woman could be in an unjustly male dominated sport. But right now, her tussle with the barbell was a perfect example of where Sonny was at. Despite her considerable driving talent, she was still depending on guts and nerve to bridge the gap between skill and the will to win. She had years to go, and miles to drive, before she gained that exquisite poise behind the wheel of the great zen road masters. But she would get there, simply because, as Lee Thomas' daughter, she would not settle for anything less. Her enduring love for her father would keep her striving to fill his shoes.

Sonny's brown eyes had softened. "Sorry about snapping at you before, but you know how I hate to fail. Anyway, Morgan, you seem to think of me as a woman at all the *wrong* times."

Morgan stared at her, wondering what in hell the kid could have meant by that. "Come on, let's lift."

He did two more sets while Sonny spotted, moving up to his best weight: ten reps at 185. Then he spotted Sonny, who, having already maxed out, did two solid sets at 110. Through it all Morgan was uneasy. He was tempted to flat out ask Sonny if she had somehow found out about his plans to expand and had been the one who had leaked the information, but he'd decided against doing that. Like Marty Robbins, if she was innocent she would be deeply offended by his accusation. Unlike Marty, she might not be so quick to forgive him for pointing the finger at her. He didn't want to lose her. She was his best test driver; and she was Lee Thomas' daughter. That alone was ample reason for him to treat her with kid gloves.

"You wanted to see me about something?" Sonny asked as she finished her last set.

She couldn't have done it, Morgan thought. She didn't even know. And yet, Sonny was the only person at DonSport with reason to hate him . . . But did *she* know that?

"You know about the Salon in Paris?" Morgan said suddenly.

"That fancy-schmancy auto show you always go to?"

"The premier automobile exhibition on the Continent," Morgan said evenly.

Sonny nodded, impatiently. "So what about it?"

"I'm leaving for Paris in a couple of days. From the Salon I'm planning to visit the Italian manufacturers whose marques we specialize in and maybe spend a little time at my place in Portofino. Anyway, I think that you ought to come along." Sonny was staring at him in astonishment. *Oh hell! She probably thinks I'm propositioning her.*

"—I mean come along to test drive the cars we might

order," Morgan hurried to add. He thought he saw something go out of her eyes, but it must have been his imagination, because Sonny seemed so very enthusiastic.

"Thank you so much! I'd love to go! You'll see, I'll be a great help on the trip, and not only test driving. I've been studying all the records and—and files—"

"You've been *what?*" Morgan demanded. *Then maybe she did know about the expansion plans.*

"Oh, shit," Sonny swallowed, backing away. "Me and my big mouth! Please don't be angry with me."

"How the hell did you get into those files?"

"I guess—well, I kind of looked at them after hours. But I only wanted to so that I could be of more help around here. I *swear* I meant well." Her smile was anxious and her voice was uncharacteristically meek. "I hope you know that?"

"What do you mean you want to be more help around here?" Morgan asked brusquely. "I thought you wanted to be a top driver?"

"I do, but I want *other* things, too." Sonny couldn't meet his eyes. "I thought, maybe, someday, I might be something like your assistant. Or maybe even a partner . . ."

Morgan let that one slide by. "I assume you have a passport?"

"Huh? Oh, sure," Sonny nodded. "I still get to go?"

"Can you be ready in a couple of days?"

"All right Morgan!" Sonny was ecstatic. "You won't regret this! You'll see what I can do!"

I just hope I haven't already *seen what you can do,* Morgan thought.

Sonny, having gathered up her racing gear, was on her way to the women's locker room. "I've got to get moving. I've got to leave early every night if I'm going to be ready, and Marty has a half-dozen more cars, and lots more tires he wants me to check out."

"Doesn't he believe in using the other drivers?"

Sonny beamed at him over her shoulder. "He believes in using the best."

"Just remember to leave a little of those cars left for the paying customers."

"Hey, somebody around here has to drive like a man," she teased, just before disappearing into the locker room.

Somebody has to drive like a man, Morgan thought. *Because I can't . . .*

The taunt had hit home. Hard. Just a joke, some vestige of rationality was pleading amidst the screech as Morgan's mind skidded out. Just a joke . . . She doesn't know; she couldn't.

And he was just paranoid. Then he remembered that today he had ample reason for paranoia. Someone had indeed betrayed him.

Suddenly Morgan found himself wondering if Sonny had actually been referring to the fact that he hadn't driven competitively since the endurance event at Le Mans when Lee Thomas crashed and burned? She knew the edited version of what had happened, but had she discovered what really went down that ended Morgan's racing career once and for all?

But that would mean that all of her friendship and enthusiasim on behalf of DonSport was just a front, an act put on to lull his suspicions.

Morgan's head was beginning to hurt again. It was all getting more hairy by the moment, and what made it worse was that Morgan didn't know how to separate the reality of what was going down from his suspicions.

Well, the reality was what he had to discover. He'd invited Sonny to come along to Europe because he'd figured the way to get her to reveal herself was to keep her close by. The thing of it was, keeping an eye on her meant that Sonny could keep an eye on him.

There were others at DonSport who might have leaked his plans, but Sonny had been his chief suspect right from the start, because she seemed to have the strongest motive: if Sonny knew the truth about her father's death, the demise of DonSport would be the least of the reprisals she would have in store for Morgan. If she were a believer in Old Testament justice, Lee Thomas' daughter would want to see Morgan dead.

6

MORGAN HAD BEEN back at his desk for a couple of hours when Beth buzzed him with the dreary news that Arthur Neal was prowling the outer office. So he gave in to the inevitable and told Beth to send him in.

Morgan was never really ready for Arthur, but he was more ready than he'd been earlier in the day. He'd returned some calls and had actually been able to get some paperwork done.

He'd also telephoned his creditors and called to make appointments with some other venture capital firms on both coasts for when he'd returned from Europe. These firms—especially the ones in New York —were less concerned with publicity than Weiner, Carlson & Boyd, and all of them had been agreeable to talking with him; but they'd also already learned that Weiner had cut him loose and that Morgan was in a tight spot. Morgan knew that these other firms would do business with him, but now that Weiner had proclaimed him damaged goods, they would demand concessions before bailing him out.

DonSport America might still happen, but at grievous financial cost to Morgan, thanks to whoever had leaked the information on his plans. Well, he'd deal with the venture capital vultures after he'd returned from Europe.

He'd settled down now that he'd invited Sonny along on his business trip. It was a move, and any move, even the wrong one, felt better than no move at all.

Now that Morgan was resigned to seeing Arthur, and now that he knew Marty Robbins had told the kid about DonSport's expansion plans, he wondered how he might get the kid to reveal if he'd been the one who leaked the information to "Viewpoint"? And what about Niles Kingman? Somebody had told him, and Arthur Neal *knew* Niles. On the other hand, Arthur Neal had no motive for betraying the company; why kill the goose laying the golden eggs?

"Mister Morgan, thank you for seeing me, sir." Arthur Neal came into the office.

"Sure, Arty. Sit down." Morgan gestured towards the grouping of chairs in front of his desk. As usual, Arthur Neal looked like he was just in from a trek down some heathered country lane. He was very into Wallabees and the Lands' End look: turtlenecks and windowpane plaids, and everything with suede elbow patches. But it looked good on him. He was in his late twenties, big and muscular, with longish, thick black wavy hair, and a square jawed, Classic Coke, captain of the football team kind of face.

"Okay, Arty, what's up?" Morgan began. "I hope work is coming along on the 969?"

Neal's dour expression brightened. "Oh yes, sir! We've been toying around with the engine, and I think I see a way to install a catalyst converter, and without castrating the car. I figure a knock sensor installed on the . . ."

Morgan put himself on cruise control; normally he paid attention to the kid's technical talk, but today he was simply too preoccupied with his own problems. Arthur Neal had made his reputation on the Grand Prix circuit, working for the Kimura/XKB-Dwyer racing team. Neal was a pioneer in the use of computers to calibrate maximum speed versus the amount of fuel being consumed. It was an important job, as each racing team is alloted a fixed quota of gas; if they run out in the middle of a race, that's their tough luck. The job was traditionally done by the team's chief mechanic, who judged the proper ratios in much the same way a master chef judges a recipe: through experience and instinct. When the Kimura-XKB car, a Japanese-British collaboration, began winning Formula One, thanks in large part to Arthur Neal's computers, the talk was that grease monkeys would soon be taking a back seat to technocrats peering into glowing green monitors as their cars raced by.

Ford was trying to lure Neal into their R&D program when Morgan approached the kid with an invitation to come head up a mini-department at DonSport. He'd offered Neal a generous salary, a staff, a research budget and free rein to tinker where his muse took him, with the provision that DonSport would take the lion's share of the profits of any breakthrough automotive whatzit that Neal might invent.

The opportunity to work free of a large corporate bureaucracy, to continue to play with exoticars, and, no doubt, to live in balmy San Francisco as opposed to rustbelt Dearborn, swayed Arthur Neal towards accepting Morgan's offer. So far, the kid had done well at DonSport, and Morgan had gotten a lot of publicity out of stealing the whiz kid away from Detroit. *"A Ford in Arthur Neal's Future? Don Morgan 'Had a Better Idea . . .'"* the *Forbes* headline had read.

"Sir?"

"Um, yeah, Arty. It sounds real good . . ." Morgan, slouched down in his seat, had swung his feet up on his desk in order to study his Nikes for wear patterns. It wasn't much of a diversion, but right now it was better than Arthur Neal's mumbo-jumbo.

"Mister Morgan, I didn't come to see you to discuss our progress on the 969. I have a problem, sir . . . It's Mister Robbins."

Morgan sighed. "Again? Why can't you guys get along?"

"I assume that is a rhetorical question, sir?"

Morgan nodded. He didn't need anyone to tell him

that he had never really considered the ramifications of bringing a hard wired technocrat into an organization managed in large part by an old-fashioned, balls-out, seat-of-the-pants type: namely, Marty Robbins. From the very first, Arthur Neal and Marty Robbins had gotten along like "Tom & Jerry" on angel dust. "What happened this time, Arty?"

"It's not any one thing, sir," Neal began. "The way the hierarchy is set up, all of my reports to you are channeled through Mister Robbins' office."

"Arty, you've got to understand that Marty is vice president in charge of R&D around here."

"You promised me that I wouldn't have to answer to anyone, Mister Morgan."

"You *don't* have to answer to Marty," Morgan reasoned. "Just show him a little respect is all I ask."

"But I don't see why I have to, sir," Neal said. "Look, Mister Morgan, I know that Mister Robbins is a friend of yours, and I guess I can understand how you might want to treat an old friend gently, the way you would a race horse or something, past its prime; I mean, you put it out to pasture, you just don't send it off to the glue factory, right?"

"Hell, I couldn't have put it better, myself," Morgan wryly agreed.

"But you've got to understand, sir; Mister Robbins isn't my friend. I mean, he's an all right old guy, but he's just not . . ." Neal hesitated.

"Say what you want to say, Arty."

Neal took a deep breath. "He's like some little kid, the way he pokes around my department, sir. He's got a million dumb questions—excuse me for saying it, sir, but they *are* dumb—and he bothers my staff, chewing their ears off about how it was done in his day, and if it was good enough for the Porsche and Mercedes racing teams, it's good enough for DonSport." Neal was leaning forward in his chair now, his fists clenched. "Well, sir, it *isn't* good enough for me. I believe in progress, I don't look back, and I'm sick of placating some backyard mechanic lost in his past by pretending that I give a rat's ass what he thinks—"

"You've built up quite a head of steam, son," Morgan tried to interject. "Just calm down."

"Don't tell me to calm down, *and stay away from Sonny!*" Arthur Neal suddenly blurted.

"Huh?" Morgan would have been less startled if the kid had pulled a .38 and begun blasting the place. He shook his head. "What the fuck are you talking about?"

"I . . . I'm sorry for speaking to you that way, sir, but I'm very upset. I . . . I saw Sonny on the way over here," Neal stammered. "She was all excited about how you were sweeping her off to Europe. We've been going together for three months, and we're good together—" Neal studied Morgan's face. "You know what I mean when I say that we're good together?"

"I get the idea," Morgan said quickly. He felt oddly disturbed by the idea of Sonny sleeping with this guy, or anyone, for that matter . . . Hell, she was certainly old enough. "Arty, I'm very glad that you and Sonny are so happy together." He wasn't happy; not at all, but he didn't want to think about that. "Please realize that I asked Sonny to come along with me to Europe for purely professional reasons."

"Take some other driver with you, then," Neal quickly challenged.

"Arty, I already asked Sonny to come, and as you know, she's accepted."

"Mister Morgan . . ." Arthur Neal blushed. "I love her, and if I thought I could prevent Sonny from going with you by proposing to her, I would. But . . ." he trailed off.

"But we both know Sonny," Morgan quietly finished for him. "So we both know that wouldn't work." Morgan smiled. "Listen to me, I swear to you that I do not have romantic intentions toward Sonny."

"She talks about you a lot, Mister Morgan," Neal said. "You mean a lot to her."

"Look, Arty, I drove with her father," Morgan said. "Now she works for me. It's only natural that she'd look up to me."

Arthur Neal stood up. "Look, Mr. Morgan, Sonny is my girl. I'm sick of competing with you for her. Maybe you didn't *know* we were in competition for her, but that doesn't change the facts. These past months, it's been difficult to work for you, harboring the resentment I feel about this."

"Have you resented me enough to spill DonSport's confidential expansion plans to the media?" Morgan demanded.

"What?" Arthur Neal looked blank.

"Marty told me how he confided in you about my plans."

Neal looked away. "Okay, I admit that I knew about your plans—"

"So it *was* you who told?"

Arthur Neal looked him right in the eye. "No, sir, it was *not* me. Mister Morgan, if I *were* going to screw you, I'd find a better way of doing it than squealing to the media. I mean, *if* I wanted to do it, I could . . . but that's beside the point. I didn't leak that information."

"Why should I believe you?" Morgan asked. "You had the means, and now I know that you had a motive."

Arthur Neal smiled coldly. "Sir, I've never had to cheat in my life. I'm the best there is in my field, and the best doesn't have to stab anybody in the back."

Morgan looked at the kid for a long moment, and then nodded. "So what's the deal, Arty. You resigning, or what?"

"Am I fired for being out of line with you, sir?"

"Of course not," Morgan replied, and then watched a slight smile play across Neal's lips. He probably takes that as a sign of weakness, Morgan brooded, and then thought, the hell with what he thinks. He's got a lot to learn about life.

"No, sir, I'm not resigning. If I did, I would no longer be working with Sonny. If I don't see you, have a very nice trip, sir."

Morgan watched Neal leave the office. Once he was alone he sank down into his chair. Doubts about people he'd thought he knew were swirling through his mind—

Marty Robbins had a motive: to get back at Morgan for hiring Arthur Neal. Arthur Neal, despite his protestations of innocence, might have leaked the information because he felt wronged about being saddled with Marty, or because of his irrational jealousy concerning Sonny—

Oh hell: and what *about* Sonny?

If what Arthur Neal had said about Sonny having a crush on him were true, it meant trouble, the kind that Morgan would have to nip in the bud. There was no way he would allow a romance to develop between himself and Lee Thomas' daughter.

Morgan's fist slammed down upon his desk top.

No way.

7

MORGAN AND SONNY landed at Orly late on a cold, drizzly night and cabbed it to the hotel. In Paris, Morgan always stayed at the Bristol. It was smaller, and more personal and discreet than either the Ritz or the Crillon, but every bit as luxurious. The cab pulled up at the Bristol's glass and wrought iron entrance, and they went inside to check in. Morgan had reserved a two bedroom suite, with separate baths and an adjoining parlor.

Upstairs, Sonny looked a little out of it; Morgan guessed the time change had caught up with her. She was wandering around the parlor with her raincoat still on, gazing dumbly at everything: the somber portraits and luminous still lifes on the wall; the trio of bowlegged, gilt-wood Louis XVI chairs, upholstered in striped satin, and grouped about a matching settee. She crossed the room to a sideboard by the windows that seemed to be sagging beneath the weight of a huge floral arrangement. "All this stuff real?" she asked.

"You mean the flowers?"

"Morgan—"

"To tell you the truth, I know that some of the furnishings are very good reproductions, but I don't know enough about antiques to say what's what." Morgan smiled. "It's real enough, though, huh?"

Sonny solemnly agreed. "My apartment is furnished with canvas backed director's chairs and pizza boxes."

Morgan steered her into a bedroom. There was a

Persian rug and a marble topped commode. The walls were covered with an ornate mirror and a pair of Boilly portraits. The bed was wide, ending in carved wooden headboard that depicted cherubs frolicking around a garland of flowers.

"It's all so beautiful," Sonny murmured as Morgan led her to the windows.

"There, to the right," he said, standing close behind her in order to peer over her shoulder through the rain streaked glass. "That tall, white, lit up deal? That's the Arc de Triomphe."

"Oh, how lovely! You know, I was just a little girl when I was here with my parents. I was really far too young to appreciate anything. We've got to go sightseeing!"

She was turned towards him now. Close enough to kiss.

Morgan stepped away. "I promise that you'll get to see everything, but it'll all still be there in the morning, so you get some rest." He closed the curtains. We've got a full day of work as well as sightseeing ahead, and a busy night. I've made dinner reservations for tomorrow at Taillevent."

"Morgan," she called to him as he left her bedroom. When he looked back he saw her pretty smile. "Thank you for bringing me. . . ."

"It's my pleasure to introduce you to nice things, Sonny," Morgan said softly. "Just as your father did for me. Sleep well."

He closed Sonny's door and then went back through the parlor to his own room: a big bed, the frilly furniture of the period, and several landscapes on the walls. He didn't have a view, but he'd seen it all before. He undressed and stretched out on the bed, thinking about what Sonny had just said to him. God, it made him feel guilty when she was being grateful to him! The irony of Sonny looking up to him the way he'd looked up to her father made him want to curl up in agony.

Morgan had meant what he'd told her. He'd been

taking care of Sonny, and Sonny's mom and sisters, for years, ever since DonSport began to turn a profit, telling Lee Thomas' widow that Lee had invested in the DonSport idea just before he died. That was a lie, of course, but one far more modest than the lie that so many people were then telling on Morgan's behalf, concerning Lee's death at Le Mans.

Morgan couldn't restore Lee Thomas to his family, but he was glad that he could at least see to it that they didn't suffer financially. Lee's widow lived comfortably in Palm Springs, and two of Lee's little girls were able to graduate from medical school thanks to those DonSport dividend checks.

When Lee's oldest daughter had shown up at DonSport, Morgan couldn't believe his eyes; couldn't believe that this was "little" Sonny Thomas sitting in his office. The last time Morgan had seen her she'd been a chubby kid.

"I love cars, and I'm good with them," Sonny had told him. "I've got some trophies to my credit. I love driving. I want it to be my life. I know you don't owe my daddy anything, but will you give me a job?"

"No, I don't owe Lee. . . ." Morgan had agreed, hating himself for how easily the lie rolled off his tongue. "When do you want to start?"

That had been two years ago. Since then Morgan had seen to it that Sonny had received every opportunity to prove herself. He had richly rewarded her successes and duly forgiven her trespasses. He supposed that a shrink would say that he was using her as a stand-in for her father; that he was trying to make it all up to Lee through Sonny. Morgan supposed the shrink would suggest that he was hoping that Lee's ghost would forgive him and stop haunting him, but Morgan already knew that could never happen.

It was still gray the next morning, with the weather report threatening sporadic drizzle. It was the way Morgan always imagined the weather in Paris: *Bogie weather.* Actually, what it was, was a lot like San Francisco weather, but it was more fun wearing a trenchcoat while wandering the Boulevard St. Michel, than the piers of Sausalito.

Morgan knocked on Sonny's closed bedroom door and called through it to tell her he'd meet her in the lobby. He then went downstairs, where he picked up a copy of the *International Tribune* to pass the time. The newspaper's front page was taken up with the usual international log jams, sprinkled with ecological disasters. Page two contained a number of articles about the current spate of art thefts, and what the European museums were doing to combat it. Morgan was about to turn the page when a sidebar piece—or rather, its byline—caught his eye. It had been written by Nicole Houel.

ART THIEVERY LINKED WITH ORGANIZED CRIME

ROME, Sept. 3. More than $100 million in art objects is stolen each year by individuals linked to organized crime, making the traffic in stolen art second only to drug dealing as the most profitable mob racket, law enforcement officials said here today.

The problem, according to the special squad of undercover police detectives assigned to investigate these crimes, is that the stolen pieces pass through the hands of so many buyers that legitimate ownership is blurred. Once the stolen piece is "laundered"—fitted with new papers and sold back into circulation—it is next to impossible for the police to track it down without an informant stepping forward.

"It used to be that people were willing to call us, because of the rewards offered for information leading to the recovery of the piece," said a police officer experienced in investigating these crimes. "Now that organized crime has gotten involved, our informants are afraid to come forward. They say that a reward isn't worth the risk of mob retribution."

England's Scotland Yard has formed a special art-theft squad, and countries such as France and Italy plan to follow that example. Overseeing and acting as a clearinghouse for these crack detective squads is Interpol, the international police organization. Interpol receives and disseminates information on stolen objets d'art, shady dealers, and art theft rings, to offices all over the world, including some countries behind the Iron Curtain. Interpol's agents are—

"Good morning!"

Morgan glanced up.

"Do I look okay?" Sonny asked, sounding nervous.

She was wearing a gray linen suit, and carrying an umbrella that matched the lining of her Burberry. Slung over her shoulder was a mammoth black leather bag crammed with yellow legal pads.

"You look like a lawyer," Morgan said, setting aside the newspaper. Sonny stared at him blankly. "But that's good," Morgan quickly added. "So where's your calculator?"

"Right here . . ." She began burrowing around in the cavernous interior of her bag. "Next to my driving shoes and gloves."

"You not only look terrific, you *are* terrific," Morgan laughed, standing up.

"Thanks, I guess," Sonny said. "But why were you so surprised?"

"I don't know," Morgan said, and then he shrugged. "Yes, I do," he admitted. "I know it isn't fair, but I can't shake my image of you the first time we met. You were what, five years old?

"Six and a half!" Sonny declared.

"You were such a chubby little thing," Morgan was shaking his head. "A regular little butterball—"

"Hey!" Sonny pirouetted before him. "Wake up and

smell the coffee, all right? You're looking at a 34-24-34!"

"Speaking of coffee—" Morgan felt compelled to change the subject. "Let's get some breakfast and get to work."

The Salon de l'Automobile Paris was being held at the National Center for Industry and Technology. It was a ruthlessly modern, concrete and glass exhibition hall in the shopping and business quarter of La Défense, which was situated twenty minutes by cab west of Paris, on the other side of the Seine, across the Pont de Neuilly. Once they'd checked in and received their credentials, Morgan sent Sonny off to explore the mega-auto show/industry convention on her own and spent the morning renewing old business contacts. He eventually linked up with Sonny at the DeManto booth. He supposed that she'd been spending a lot of time there, but then that did make a kind of sense. *Like father, like daughter,* Morgan thought to himself.

"Hi!" Sonny handed Morgan a sheaf of notes. "I've covered all the Europeans, with the exception of the Italian firms, because I figured you'd want to handle them yourself."

Morgan glanced at her notes. They were clear and complete, right down to technical specifications. She had even gotten the anticipated lengths of time needed for stateside delivery. He checked her price notations. He read them twice. "Sonny, I think you got these prices wrong. They look very low."

"They're correct," she said.

"But how?"

"Not bad for a butterball," she bragged. "I got one manufacturer to take fifteen percent off; then I told the other manufacturers about it, and they all fell into line in order to stay competitive. It was easy!" She laughed excitedly. "I love this, Morgan! You should have seen them! They just about fell over themselves to offer cars to us. They all want American movie stars driving their cars. Thanks to your Hollywood connections, DonSport has a lock on what the manufacturers think is a very elite, trend setting market."

"I'm very pleased," Morgan told her. He held up the notes. "This is as thorough a job as I could have done. It's going to save me a lot of time. You've certainly learned a lot about the business . . ."

"You sound surprised."

"I guess I am, a little bit," Morgan admitted. "I just never knew you were so capable off of the race track."

"I guess there's a lot about me you don't know," she said soberly.

That stopped Morgan short. Just how much about her didn't he know? That she was the one who leaked the information?

"Why are you looking at me so funny?" Sonny asked.

"Hmm? Oh, no reason." Morgan forced a smile. "What's next on your agenda?"

"They've set up a small test loop out behind the hall. I thought I'd test drive a couple of new models. Is that all right?"

"Sure . . ." Morgan said absently, as suspicions about Sonny, *and* Marty Robbins, *and* Arthur Neal, again began to torment him.

"Morgan? Are you okay?" Sonny asked, studying him. "You look like you ate a bad escargot."

He glanced at his watch. "Meet you back here in two hours," Morgan said. "Don't forget that we've got some sightseeing to do before we go back to the hotel to change for dinner."

"Can we?" Sonny pleaded. "Will we have time?"

"Thanks to you, we will," Morgan assured her. "I meant it when I said your notes are going to save me a lot of running around. You've more than earned your keep on this trip."

Morgan spent a quarter hour negotiating with the DeManto people about the company's new, turbocharged, full-time, four wheel drive convertible, the

Gatto. The production run was a scant 200 for the two hundred thousand dollar automobile, and all of those had already been spoken for. Morgan convinced them to manufacture twenty more for DonSport, and to take another five percent off the total shipment price for old time's sake. In return he promised the DeManto exec that he'd take one of the prototypes for a spin around the test loop out back and then submit to a publicity photo session. Morgan then perused Sonny's notes and went over to see the Courser-Anton people. That British firm was also producing an exclusive, limited run, ultra-high-performance car for the upcoming season. Morgan purchased ten, even though the company exec wouldn't budge below the already excellent discount Sonny had sweet-talked him into. Morgan figured that if he didn't immediately sell these cars, or the DeManto four wheel drives, these one-chance-only series vehicles would only appreciate in value.

It was time to head over to the test loop to keep his appointment with the DeManto execs. The clouds had begun to break, and the sun was peeking through as Morgan left the exhibition hall, and took a shuttle bus to the section of La Défense's ring road barricaded off for test drives and photo opportunities. The DeManto execs, along with a flock of photographers, were waiting near the signature red Gatto, its tan soft top up against the uncertain weather. In the roped off section next door, Morgan saw Sonny hiking up her gray skirt to flash an enticing length of thigh as she swung herself behind the wheel of a Maserati. Morgan waved to her, but she didn't notice him. It didn't surprise him. When Sonny was around cars, she was all business.

Morgan posed beside the Gatto, and then behind the wheel for a few pictures, then started up the big, V-12 engine, and guided the DeManto out onto the roadway. The car's clutch made Morgan glad he'd not neglected his Nautilus lower body exercises, and the steering was equally heavy. He thought the Gatto was excessively noisy, and it didn't accelerate at quite the DeManto trademark warp-drive velocity. That was likely due to the extra weight of the four wheel drive hardware. On the plus side, the driver's seat was exceptionally comfortable, and the ergonomically designed instruments and controls were a joy to use. The full time, four wheel drive made the car feel like it was glued to the road, even *this* road, still rain-slick. A pesky tendency to fishtail during less than ideal road conditions, or during some aggressive driving maneuvers, had always been the Achilles heel of the nimble and powerful DeMantos. With the Gatto that problem had been eradicated, making this vehicle as perfect a sports car as any ultrawealthy road warrior could hope to own.

Morgan drove a few laps on the largely deserted roadway, and then brought the car back. As he pulled into the parking area he was surprised to see Nicole Houel talking with some of the DeManto execs. She looked smashing in baggy, green tweed slacks, and one of those brown leather *Raiders of the Lost Ark* style jackets. Morgan spent a few minutes chatting with some of the DeManto technicians about the Gatto and posed for a few final pictures. By then, Nicole had concluded her interview, and he went over.

"This is a coincidence," Morgan said. "I saw your article in today's *Tribune*, and now here you are."

"I applied for my press credentials months in advance," she laughed, kissing him on the cheek. "I wouldn't have missed this for the world. I like fast cars, and fast men." Her big green eyes locked on his. She looked mystified. "But I noticed that you weren't driving very fast at all."

"I never do, on a track." Morgan smiled. "The truth is, I'm scared to death of race tracks."

"You're making fun of me, now," Nicole chided. "Do you intend to do any more driving?"

"Nope. I'm all done."

Nicole slipped her arm through his. "Then let's steal away. Come, you'll buy me a chocolate to warm me, yes? I adore chocolate, and there's a cafe nearby."

As they strolled away from the driving area Sonny came past in the Maserati. The car slowed, and Morgan thought he saw Sonny staring in his direction, but before he could be sure, the Maserati picked up speed and roared away.

It was coming on lunch time, so the large cafe, on the plaza adjoining the CNIT Hall, was bustling. Its decor was "Old Parisian," right down to the obligatory zinc topped bar, which meant that the cafe had to have been as carefully assembled as a stage set since the joint couldn't be any older than the rest of the La Défense complex, which had been built sometime in the sixties.

"Let's find a table," Nicole shouted into Morgan's ear, once they were through the door and in the midst of the din. He nodded and began elbowing his way through the business suited bar crowd in order to get them to the table section at the rear. Once they were past the crush, Nicole took the lead. She seemed to be heading someplace in particular, so Morgan followed, past the cafe's inset mirrors and ceramic tiled walls.

Nicole stopped at a table already occupied by Niles Kingman, florid of countenance, wearing a Stetson, and smoking a foot long cigar.

"This was just a setup?" Morgan frowned. "Nicole, why are you birddogging for this guy?"

"I did ask Nicole to bring you here," Kingman said. He stood up and offered his hand. He was wearing jeans, a plaid flannel shirt, and an ultrasuede sports jacket to go along with his cowboy hat. Morgan struggled against the urge to whistle a few bars of "An American in Paris."

"Niles needed to see you," Nicole began, "So I—"

"And all this time I thought it was my animal magnetism," Morgan cut her off.

"Don't be angry with me," she pleaded.

"I'm not angry, just baffled," Morgan said. "What's going on?"

"I do apologize for the subterfuge," Kingman said. "But I figured that if I tried to corner you over at the convention hall you'd duck me. But who could duck a looker like Nicole here, eh?"

"She is unduckable," Morgan agreed.

"Anyway, I figure this here's a much more private kind of place for us to talk; there's just too many people hanging around the exhibition hall." Kingman sat back down. "You see, Morgan, I intend to make you a business proposition."

"If you have something to say I'll certainly listen," Morgan shrugged.

"Then sit down," Kingman grinned, settling back in his chair. "Hey!" he bellowed at a passing waiter. "You there! *Garçon!*"

Nicole sighed, and glanced at Morgan as he pulled out a chair for her.

"Hold on, there, darlin'," Kingman said pleasantly. He shook his head. "This is private," he told Nicole. "So why don't you just run along, and do some writin' or shoppin' or somethin'."

Nicole hesitated, clearly not wanting to leave, but Kingman stared her down. She nodded to him, whispered to Morgan, "I'm at the Hôtel du Carrousel. Call me," and went off.

Niles puffed contentedly on his cigar. A poker-faced waiter came over, and Morgan ordered espresso.

"That's quite a getup," Morgan commented.

"'Dallas' is very popular over here. Maybe everybody thinks you're J.R."

"Say what?"

Morgan shook his head. "Not important. You said you had some business to discuss with me?"

Kingman leaned back in his chair. "I do. I heard that Weiner faded on you after 'Viewpoint' went public with your plans."

"Stop there," Morgan interrupted. "I've been wondering, how *did* you happen to know about my plans when we talked together at Grace Tyler's wedding? That was hours before 'Viewpoint' aired . . ."

Kingman winked. "Morgan, when you spend as much money on TV advertising as we do, you develop your media sources. Some days earlier, an account executive from one of the local stations we do business with got advance look at the 'Viewpoint' tape for that week's broadcast. The guy called me, thinking that the information would be to my advantage." He smiled broadly. "And it was . . ."

"How so?"

"You still interested in going nationwide with DonSport?" Kingman asked.

"Sure."

"Well, you should be," Kingman nodded, "'cause it's a good idea. So good, as a matter of fact, that we—my dad and I—are interested in seein' it to fruition."

Morgan forced himself to surpress his excitement. His guts told him that he could cut a better deal with Kingman than he could with any of those investment firms waiting in the wings to fight over his bones. He was very aware of Kingman watching him. He began to fiddle with his espresso, stirring it, rubbing the itty-bitty lemon peel around the rim of the itty-bitty cup. He put sugar into the espresso and stirred it some more, and he didn't even *like* sugar in his espresso. What he couldn't do was allow Niles to catch on to his almost desperate eagerness.

"We'd like to take over where Weiner left off," Kingman drawled. He hooked his thumbs behind his beaded belt's brass buckle. It looked substantial enough to stop a bullet.

"Let me get this straight. You're talking about financing my expansion?" When Kingman nodded, Morgan continued. "And you've already gotten your father's blessings on this?"

"Dad thinks it's a great idea," Kingman said. "Assumin' we can come to mutually agreeable terms, of course."

"Do you realize what kind of money you're talking about?" Morgan asked warily.

Kingman studied the backs of his manicured nails. "Not as much as you probably think," he said. "Leastways, not nearly as much as you needed from Weiner. You were likely figuring on building your dealerships from the ground up, or maybe taking over suitable, vacant, *existing* locations to house your operations; am I right?"

Morgan nodded. "Weiner and I triple-checked the numbers, and we couldn't find a way to go nationwide with outlets in a handful of key locations for under twelve mill."

"But Kingman and Son already *have* the retail outlets for you," Kingman pointed out. "And it's a hell of a lot more than a handful of locations. What we're offering you is the opportunity to sell DonSport vehicles out of our dealerships. We're sorta thinking along the lines of the relationship that, say, Caroll Shelby has enjoyed with Ford and Chrysler.

"No offense, Niles, but I've never had partners, and I'm not sure I want any now."

Kingman held up his hands. His fingernails glinted, his gold bracelet and watch gleamed, and his diamond pinkie ring sparkled. Paris at night didn't throw off so much light. "No offense, buddy, but Dad and I don't want partners, *ever*. What I'm talking about here is strictly a leasing arrangement. A lot of our dealerships have showrooms and maintenance areas lying idle, or, at least, not earning back our investment to full potential. We'd rent that showroom space to you, and bill you for your use of the garage facilities, simple as that."

"And my start-up costs?" Morgan asked.

"We'd have to sit and talk specific numbers," Kingman cautioned, "but, in general, we're prepared to finance—let's say for now—half of your start-up costs."

"And that would be a loan?" Morgan asked. "You'd be lending money to DonSport, not buying a piece of it?"

"A loan." Kingman nodded. "I'm sure we can work out mutually agreeable terms. You'll have to come up with the rest of your funding on your own, but don't forget that we've eliminated your real estate costs. We're now talkin' about a small fraction of the sum you discussed with Weiner."

Morgan looked at him. It was funny how an interesting business proposition could change your attitude about a guy. . . . He had to admit he was very intrigued by Kingman's proposal. He didn't like Niles' business reputation, but had the highest regard for his father, Sam Kingman. If Sam was for the deal, it had to be on the up-and-up.

Anyway, Morgan was looking for financing, and Kingman was looking to deal. Any port in a storm.

"So far we've discussed what I get out of this," Morgan said. "What's in it for you and your father?"

Kingman's broad, freckled countenance split into another of his Chesire cat grins. "Hell, we get *class!* The thing of it is, Dad and I make a mint peddlin' econoboxes, and here and there in urban areas we got us a Mercedes dealership, but that don't get us diddlysquat in the prestige and respect departments."

"So what you're negotiating for is the right to use my name and reputation as a blanket endorsement of your operations."

"Why not, Morgan? Check us out, if you want. Call the Better Business Bureau any place we operate. We're fuckin' squeaky clean as the Boy Scouts. My dad wouldn't have it any other way."

Morgan nodded. "I know that your father is as honest as they come, Niles—and I'm sure that you've followed in his footsteps," he thought to hastily add.

"I can see the media campaign now." Kingman's

jewelry encrusted hands wrote in the air. *"Donnie Morgan chose Kingman and Son because of our reputation. So should you!"* He winked. "Of course, if we do this deal, we're gonna want more than just the right to use your name."

"Like a part of the net profits?" Morgan asked.

Kingman's thumb and index finger rubbed together. "A li'l tiny piece," he consoled. "To be negotiated later. Believe me, Morgan, we're comin' to *you* on this. We're flexible. We're not lookin' for deal breakers, here."

"I've got some conditions," Morgan said.

"Name 'em."

"Number one, I hire my own people to staff my operations."

"Hire who you want," Kingman shrugged. "Our salespeople are used to dicking around with the customers over the cost of the floormats. They don't know shit from shinola about selling hundred grand and up cars. But I've got to insist that you transport your cars from U.S. port of entry to the dealerships using our existing delivery subsidiary corporation; otherwise, you're going to cause us union problems. While those cars are in transit, my delivery people will be in charge of 'em, otherwise my insurance will skyrocket. Once the cars are at the actual retail sales outlet, your DonSport personnel can take over. Fair enough?"

Morgan nodded. "Number two, if your organization wants any piece of my action it's going to have to take the bitter with the sweet. If you know so much, you know that I'm over-extended optioning real estate I no longer need. We're going to have to do a sidebar deal to let me get DonSport out of hock. Finally, I'll want you to absorb a to-be-negotiated-but-substantial portion of my legal costs when the North American Alliance of Foreign Auto Dealers decides to sue my ass."

Kingman laughed. "No problem on the side deal, or the legal stuff. We got lawyers and lobbyists on retainer with nothing to do but play with their secretarys' tits.

Let NAAFAD scream their fuckin' heads off if they want. Kingman and Son didn't get to be where it is today by being afraid to step on a few toes."

"Well, then," Morgan smiled, thinking his gut reaction about Kingman had been accurate. "It's starting to sound very good to me."

"There is one li'l thing . . ." Kingman drawled. "What I got in mind is a publicity stunt designed to get this new operation of ours hitting the ground running. What I propose is a race at Le Mans."

"What?"

"A li'l 'mini-race' just a couple of hours long," Kingman elaborated, "between all the manufacturers that DonSport now—or will—represent. The manufacturers wouldn't have to do anything but enter the same cars you'd be selling."

"You're talking about street cars; totally unmodified; just the way they are when they come out of the factory?" Morgan asked.

"That's right. We'll keep it simple, so that the race can take place real soon."

Morgan thought about it. "I don't know if the manufacturers would go for it. Some of them might worry about the potential for public humiliation when their cars are stacked up against the competition."

"Hell, we could structure the damned race so that everybody wins something, just to keep everyone happy, like at a damned kid's birthday party. Kingman and Son would pay the costs of running the event."

Morgan nodded slowly. "I hear you. You know, there's something like what you're talking about, that takes place in the United States."

"There you go," Kingman enthused.

"I think the SCCA, the Sports Car Club of America, runs it. I'll check it out with some SCCA officials I know." Morgan grinned. "Niles, it's not a bad idea."

"It's a great idea!" Kingman insisted. "And the press will eat it up. I know they will, because I already talked to Nicole about it. She's anxious to handle the media for us on this."

"She is?"

"Yep," Kingman grinned slyly. "You'd be workin' real close with her on this, Morgan. I hope that won't be too much of a hardship on you."

"I'd think the hardship, in that case, would be yours, Niles," Morgan replied quietly.

"Nah—Nicole and me are just good buddies," Kingman said. "Ain't nothin' more than some good times in the sack between us." He waved aside the entire conversation, as if it were too trivial to concern himself with. "So what d'ya say about my race idea?"

"If you're willing to underwrite the costs of the event, I think I could convince the manufacturers to take part," Morgan mused. "There's no logistical problem, as the cars are all already here in Paris, and it's just a few hours, by truck, to Le Mans. There's nothing doing at Le Mans now, so arranging for the use of the facilities shouldn't be a problem."

"Here's the kicker," Kingman smiled. "After the race, all of these state-of-the-art performance cars get sent to American to make a tour of the Kingman and Son dealerships in order to drum up free advance publicity for the coming DonSport outlets. What d'ya think of *that?*"

"I think that we might have to buy those cars to pry them loose from the companies that own them. We're talking about several million dollars worth of vehicles."

"So we buy 'em if we have to," Kingman shrugged. "From here on, several mill is gonna be petty cash for you, Morgan," he said expansively. "Anyway, I bet'cha we don't have to buy 'em. Now that you're with Kingman and Son, you'll be one of the biggest foreign car distributors in America. These here manufacturers will all bend over and spread for you, don't you worry 'bout that. Take it from one who knows, when you're a big boy, everybody else gets out of your way."

"In that case, I think we have the makings of a deal," Morgan smiled. He extended his hand across the table, but Kingman made no move to take it.

"Of course, you'll drive in this mini Le Mans," Kingman added. "You gettin' back behind the wheel in an honest-to-god race will *really* make headlines. Yep," Kingman was nodding to himself, "if we're to get maximum media play—I'm talking 'Entertainment Tonight,' the Carson/Letterman circuit, the whole damn smear—you've *got* to drive in that race."

When hell freezes over, Morgan thought. "Sure, I'll drive. We have a deal," he smiled brightly, and he and Niles Kingman shook hands.

8

MORGAN AND SONNY spent the rest of what turned out to be a lovely day sightseeing. Morgan didn't mind doing all those tourist things, because he was having such a great time re-experiencing Paris through Sonny's unjaded eyes.

As the sun set they returned to the Bristol to rest for a couple of hours, and then dressed for dinner at Taillevent. Sonny, radiant in a strapless, satin banded black dress, was awestruck from the moment they arrived at the gray, stone building on the Rue Lamennais, a street which had always reminded Morgan of the staid, monied, residential blocks of New York's East Side. As they passed through the restaurant's large glass doors, Morgan was warmly greeted by the maître d', and the proprietor, and then scolded for staying away for so long. Morgan spent a few moments chatting with the gentlemen in his awkward French, and then he and Sonny were seated at his favorite table in the softly lit, oak paneled, back dining room Morgan preferred.

"Did you understand what everyone was saying to you?" Sonny murmured once they were seated.

"I didn't even understand what I was saying," Morgan shrugged. "When it comes to French, if I can't eat it, I can't pronounce it."

"They seemed to understand you."

"They always can, if they like you," he muttered.

"Didn't my dad used to say that?" Sonny asked, amused.

Morgan grinned. He reached across the table to take her hand. "I'm very glad you're here."

"Are you really?" She sighed contentedly, looking like a princess in the lambent light cast by the candelabra wall sconces. "I thought I was embarrassing you. I mean, everyone is looking at me."

"I noticed it, too," Morgan replied, smiling.

"What am I doing wrong?" Sonny implored.

"Honey, don't you know admiring glances when you see them?" It was true. Taillevent's clientele were some of the most chic and sophisticated people in Paris, and they were sneaking looks at Sonny as if they were going to beg her for an autograph at any moment. "I guess they know a winner when they see one," Morgan added, and suddenly flashed on how this was just how it used to be with Ilsa.

"Can we have champagne?" Sonny asked.

"We can have anything we want," Morgan was happy to be able to say. As he gazed at Sonny the painful memories of Ilsa faded, until all that was left was his pleasure and pride in being in the company of a beautiful woman.

Morgan conferred with the sommelier and then had him bring a bottle of Piper Rare 76 for Sonny.

They ordered oysters poached with white leeks, and cloudlike, seafood quenelles floating in a butter sauce studded with bits of black truffles to start, followed by salad. There was a lemon sorbet, and then sliced breast of duck in black current sauce for Sonny, while Morgan had baby lamb chops. Morgan suggested another wine to accompany Sonny's main course, but she was very happy to continue drinking champagne. During the leisurely meal Morgan carefully steered the conversation away from business. They talked about the beauty of Paris, and what they would see in Italy when they arrived there, the day after tomorrow. It wasn't until they were being served coffee that Morgan brought up his conversation with Niles Kingman. "By the way, it looks as if DonSport is going to go national, after all . . ."

He kept a careful eye on her as he outlined the tentative deal, wondering if she'd reveal her true feelings by showing consternation over the fact that his plans had not been permanently shelved by the "Viewpoint" news leak. His purely paternal fondness for her aside, he still couldn't completely trust her. Sure, their affection for each other seemed strong, but Morgan could never forget the fact that their entire relationship was founded on a lie. His lie, he guiltily reminded himself. For both their sakes, he hoped he could keep his lie intact. If Sonny were to find out the truth, their friendship would surely crumble.

And if she already knew the truth? Well, she was one hell of an actress if she were concealing her animosity. *Okay, what if she were one hell of an actress?*

". . . Anyway, what Kingman has suggested is pretty much a basic leasing of his existing space, and a co-op use of his garage facilities," Morgan finished up. "I'd buy the specialized equipment each outlet would require to maintain the cars we handle," he shrugged. "If I go through with it, that is . . ."

Morgan had purposely cast the deal in the worst possible terms. He was playing devil's advocate in order to draw Sonny out. He wanted to discover how much she had learned about his business in general. So far, he'd been very impressed by her. If it turned out that she was innocent of betraying him, of course . . .

Sonny was looking uncomfortable. "I've been hesitant to discuss any of this with you . . . I mean, from going through the files, I knew about your plans to expand." She thought it over. "I guess you'd have to call them *stymied* plans, since the 'Viewpoint' broadcast. Anyhow, I've done some thinking—" she paused, blushing. "Research, I guess you'd have to call it, in case we ever had this conversation, but you never brought it up, and I was afraid to; I figured it was too touchy."

"Okay," Morgan nodded. "So now I've brought it up, and I'm asking for some feedback."

"In that case, I think it's a great idea," Sonny declared. "And I don't understand why you're so hesitant."

"A couple of reasons," Morgan said. "One of them is that I'm concerned that we'll lose our aura of exclusivity. We pretty much do sell the sizzle rather than the steak, you know. Will our clientele think twice about spending a hundred grand plus for an automobile from the same facility that sells Toyotas?"

"I've got some input on that," Sonny said.

Morgan laughed. "That's an Arthur Nealism, if I've ever heard one," he blurted, and immediately regretted his remark, cursing himself for having totally forgotten that Arthur Neal and Sonny were romantically involved. "Sonny, what I meant was—"

"Excuse me, but how did you know that Arthur and I are seeing each other?"

"Uh, um, I didn't. I mean—"

"Morgan, don't lie. You *do* know. I can tell you do, by the way you began blushing as soon as you mentioned Arthur's name. Right now you can't even look me in the eye. "Did Artie tell you? Is that how you found out?"

"Yeah, Artie told me," Morgan confessed. "I guess you know that he was a little upset by the fact that you were coming with me on this trip."

"Really?" Sonny grinned.

"Oh, shit," Morgan groaned.

"Don't take it so hard," Sonny told him. "You haven't told me anything I couldn't have guessed on my own. Artie tries to play it cool, but I know how he really feels; he loves me."

"That's a—very nice," Morgan stuttered, feeling supremely uncomfortable.

"Do you want to know how I feel about Artie?"

"Sonny, I'm really very happy for both of you," Morgan gamely plodded on. "I feel very much like a father towards you, honey, and I want you to know that you can always turn to me for—"

"I don't love Artie," Sonny interrupted. "Would you like to know who I do love?" She paused. "Or would you like to get back to discussing business?"

"You play much poker?" Morgan grumbled. "You ought to."

"I'm still waiting for your answer," Sonny said sweetly.

"Yes," Morgan nodded, and then shook his head. "I mean, I'd be interested in hearing your input; in getting back to business." He was very aware of Sonny's pretty brown eyes upon him.

"Well, okay," she said slowly, smiling.

"What is so funny?" Morgan challenged.

"Private joke. And that's all I'll say about it. Don't forget, you're the one who is insisting we talk business. "Let's see, before I begin, keep in mind that I've got most of this written down back home, but here's what I can remember, which is probably not very much after three glasses of champagne. Everything I'm about to say is based on the supposition that the DonSport outlets will be selling only the *crème de la crème*." She glanced at a nearby waiter. "I'd better keep my voice down. You can probably order *crème de la crème* in a place like this."

"Sonny, quit stalling."

"I am stalling, aren't I?" She took a deep breath and let it out. "Sorry, but I feel like this is my big chance, and I'm afraid I'll blow it."

"Don't worry," Morgan softly told her. "You won't ever run out of chances with me."

"You mean it?"

"I do," he said, realizing that he really did. Even if she *had* been the one who betrayed him, he'd still forgive her. She was Lee Thomas' daughter, and nothing she could do to him could ever equal the wrong he'd done Lee.

"Okay, what I meant about the *crème* business is that we'd sell only the top-of-the-line, new and used Eurocar exotics: Ultra-status cars the client will find nowhere else, especially not with the kinds of warranties and maintenance contracts that DonSport offers, and *double especially* not in the usual dealer showrooms.

"We've never really gotten into the used market before," Morgan said doubtfully.

"Sure we have, we just called them *vintage, refurbished,* and so on," Sonny pointed out. "Anyway, I think we'll have to get into it in order to snare that share of the market who has only, say, forty thousand or so to spend on a car. We want that individual—that person who can be persuaded that there is more inherent status in an exotic marque as opposed to the latest in high tech—to come to us for a vintage DeManto as opposed to going elsewhere for a new Porsche. Don't forget that when we go nationwide with Kingman and Son, we won't be selling mostly to celebrities, like we are now."

"That's *if* we go nationwide with the Kingmans," Morgan corrected her.

"Morgan, I worked out the figures. I just *know* that with the right guidance each outlet could do between nine and thirteen million a year," she said devoutly.

"You still haven't addressed my concerns about the loss of prestige we'll suffer sharing space with ordinary dealerships."

"I think you're overestimating the extent of that problem," Sonny replied earnestly. "The prosperous people who buy our kind of cars are looking for a symbol of their success. They've worked hard, and want a toy that makes it all worthwhile; a toy they can enjoy and flaunt. That toy is the *car*, Morgan. It's not where they *bought* it." She winked. "The *car* is the star; the rest of it is like that star's dressing room. Nobody cares about where the ownership papers get signed, or where the oil gets changed."

"Some people might," Morgan argued. "Some might expect the best technical support available to backup that major a purchase."

"Okay, you're right," Sonny admitted. "But that sort of person can only respond positively to the DonSport nameplate being on the back of their prospective vehicle. They'll know—because we'll tell them —that the DonSport tradition, forged over the years at the San Francisco facility, has carried over to the outlet where they're buying their car. The DonSport nameplate is a status symbol in itself. It proclaims to the world that the owner of this vehicle was savvy enough and rich enough to buy a high performance car at a premier, high performance sales outlet. Who gives a shit if over at the other side of the building somebody else is selling a Toyota? You can park a DeManto right *next* to a Toyota, but there's still a hell of a difference between the two. The same goes for the dealership. Just because the two dealerships share a physical space doesn't mean they're the same."

Morgan was pleased that Sonny could so positively put her finger on what really made his business tick. "You know, a lot of what you're saying could be the basis of our inaugural advertising campaign."

She barely smiled, but her almond eyes were alight, and only part of it had to do with the flickering candles. "That thought has crossed my mind." She was watching him eagerly, now. "Does that mean we're going to go through with it?"

She *couldn't* have betrayed me, Morgan thought. If Sonny's enthusiasm about the business was fake, then he was Mario Andretti. "It means I'm very *close* to agreeing to the deal," he said. "There are still a few minor points I have to iron out with Niles Kingman, and one little point I have to iron out with you."

"Which is?"

Morgan filled her in on Kingman's idea for kicking

111

off the DonSport America promotional campaign with a mini-race at Le Mans. Sonny seemed upset when Morgan mentioned that Nicole Houel would be acting as the official liaison to the media.

"That would be the busty redhead you went off with this afternoon?" Sonny frowned.

"As a matter of fact, yeah, it is," Morgan said. "You know her?"

"No, but when I saw you two go off together this afternoon, I asked around. Why does *she* have to be involved?" Sonny complained. "There's plenty of public relations types who could do a better job than *her*. What's *she* got going for her, beyond T-and-A, I mean?"

"She's a friend of Niles, and I guess he wanted to throw some work her way," Morgan said.

"She's Niles' friend?" Sonny asked, sounding somewhat mollified.

"Yes," Morgan said, truthfully.

"Not yours? I mean, there's nothing between the two of you?"

"No, of course not," Morgan lied through his teeth, all the while wondering why he felt the need to?

"That's okay, then, I guess," Sonny said slowly.

"Anyway, what I wanted to talk over with you concerns the race at Le Mans," Morgan said. "I've been thinking about what you mentioned to me back in San Francisco: that you were interested in scaling back on racing, and moving into a management position at DonSport. Do you still feel that way?"

"You know that I do."

"Good, because if this deal with Kingman works out, I've decided to put you in charge of our expanded dealership network."

Sonny laughed excitedly. "I feel like I'm dreaming! I appreciate your confidence in me, and I promise you that I won't let you down."

"I'm sure you won't." Okay, Morgan thought. The

hook is set, and now it's time to reel her in. He felt like a heel. "Sonny, there's a catch."

She nodded wryly. "I guess there always is. Although I must say, I'm intrigued. That line coming from some other guy would start me thinking that I'm expected to sleep my way into the job."

"Sonny." Morgan was appalled. "It's not like *that*."

She laughed affectionately. "God, how could anybody who's been around as much as you, have stayed so straight?"

Morgan ignored the question. "One thing I've learned about this line of work is that you need charisma to succeed. It helps when people want to meet you just to say they shook your hand. Along that line, I was thinking of hiring a more accomplished ex-driver for this job, or even an athlete from some totally unrelated sport."

"I see, you're worried that people are going to say 'who?' when I call them up." Sonny shrugged. "I don't know what to say to that, beyond that I'll do my best for you, and if I knew how to get famous, I'd do it."

"I know a way for you to get famous," Morgan said. "It has to do with the publicity race at Le Mans. I'm supposed to drive in that race. Niles Kingman, and everyone else thinks I'm going to, but I'm not. You are."

Sonny stared at him. "That's impossible. It wouldn't be allowed. The manufacturers would withdraw their support before they let a woman drive at Le Mans."

"They'd quit if they knew about it beforehand," Morgan pointed out. "But they're not going to know about it until it's over and done."

"You want to substitute me in your place, without telling anyone?" she asked skeptically.

"We could pull it off, Sonny," Morgan insisted. "Think about it."

"I am, and it seems totally impossible—"

"Why?" Morgan reasoned. "You're about my

height. Picture yourself suited up in bulky racing gear, wearing a helmet. With all the activity going on, nobody is going to look at you twice as you get into the car." He was talking fast, now; not pausing for breath, afraid to let her get a word in edgewise in his rush to convince her. "I'll give my interviews before the race, and then go in to change. I stay in, and you come out, suited up, with that helmet on. Everyone will keep their distance; nobody disturbs a driver in the moments before a race. You get into the car, and there you go."

She'd been watching him intently all through this spiel. "Morgan, why don't you want to drive in this race?"

She really doesn't know the truth about me, Morgan decided, looking into her concerned eyes. And if she doesn't know why I can't drive, she doesn't know about what really happened concerning her father, which means she would have had no reason to betray me by leaking information to "Viewpoint."

He guessed that he had already pretty much reached that conclusion; he just hadn't consciously admitted it to himself. His case against her had begun to unravel from the moment they'd arrived in Paris. She'd been behaving all along in a manner that was just too ingenuously sincere. He'd bet his life that she wasn't a backstabber . . . Come to think of it, he *was* betting his life.

"You haven't answered my question," she softly repeated. "You haven't participated in a race since my father died. Why is that?"

He was just *this* close to telling her, but the words, formed over a decade ago during countless, shame-filled, sleepless nights, stuck in his throat. He had seen enough death in his life, and so he feared and dreaded the day when Sonny might learn the truth, and her affection toward him evaporate. He would postpone that awful moment for as long as he could, and especially for now. Regardless of whether Sonny was friend or foe, she was on this night a divinely lovely being, and he did not want to see the radiance die in her almond eyes, to be replaced by that same repugnance he felt toward himself.

"You've got it all wrong," Morgan forced himself to laugh. "I was going to race, honestly I was, but then I got this idea concerning you, that's all. Imagine the pandemonium when you drive into the winners' circle and pull off your helmet. You'll be an instant *mega-*celebrity—"

"What I'll be is disqualified," Sonny complained.

"So what? It's an unofficial race. A publicity stunt. And no matter what they claim, they can't wipe away the reality of the fact that you won."

"I might not win."

"I think you will," Morgan said. "I know you, and I know how you drive. But say you don't. It's virtually a certainty that you'll place. You'll still gain the kind of instant celebrity needed to do the job for DonSport."

Sonny was subdued. "If I do this, it's going to cause a lot of hard feeling against me in the racing establishment. I'd probably end up blackballed right the hell out of the sport."

Morgan stared at her. He didn't know what to say.

"That hadn't occurred to you?"

It hadn't. Morgan felt awful. When Niles Kingman had made Morgan's participation in the race a necessity if their deal was to go through, Morgan had latched onto the idea of substituting Sonny for himself without really thinking through the ramifications to her driving career. The racing establishment was tradition bound and could be very vindictive towards rebels, upstarts, wavemakers.

"I guess you have to make a decision, Sonny," Morgan said sincerely.

"You mean if I don't drive in the race, I don't get the job?"

"Like I said, I want somebody with clout in that position. You have to decide what's most important to you." He was being an asshole for putting her in this spot, but he didn't know what else to do. Somebody had to drive for him in this damned race Kingman had his heart set on. There was no way Morgan could drive in competition. He'd tried it once, after Lee Thomas' death. He'd been off the booze for six months, and figured he was ready to get it up for a nothing, little, SCCA sponsored amateurs' race, but he never even got the lilliputian Formula Vee into gear. He just sat there in the pit, turned to jelly behind the wheel. He'd been shaking so badly that he'd needed help to get out of the car. He'd never forget the awful humiliation. . . .

"Morgan, are you all right?" Sonny asked, concerned.

He shook himself. "I'm fine." It took as much effort as he had ever expended in the gym, pumping iron, to pretend that he was. "I was thinking. I'm sorry."

"You were a thousand miles away, all right," Sonny agreed.

He'd let the deal with Kingman fall through before he again humiliated himself, trying, and failing, to drive in a race, Morgan decided. If Sonny didn't drive for him, he'd let the deal fall through.

"Morgan, the job you're offering me is very important; I know that, and I'm grateful." Sonny paused. "But racing means a lot to me, too. You being who you are, and having known my father, can understand that . . . I guess what I'm asking for is some time to think all of this over," Sonny said.

Morgan nodded. "I'll tell you what: I'm not going to do anything about the race until we get to Italy. I'm going to make my initial pitch to Professor DeManto. If the old man goes for it, chances are most of the other Italian marques will fall into line. If I can get all or most of the Italians to enter, the other manufacturers will have to go along, unless they want to look like they're afraid to compete. You take these next couple of days to sort out your priorities."

* * *

It was a lovely night as they left the restaurant; it was cool, but there was no wind, and the velvety, midnight blue sky was perfectly clear. They bundled up in their coats and walked the short distance to the broad, glittering Champs Elysées, and then strolled to the Arc de Triomphe, luminously pale in the night-turned-to-day glare of its flood lights.

They were quiet during their walk, and during the cab ride back to the Bristol. Morgan guessed that both of them were preoccupied with their thoughts. Upstairs, in their suite, Morgan told Sonny to "sleep tight," and headed for his own bedroom.

"Stay up a little longer," Sonny begged, kicking off her black pumps and curling up on the sofa.

"Sonny, it's late. We've got work to do tomorrow."

"Oh, I know," she sighed. "But today has been so lovely; so exciting and eventful; I don't want the night to end. I swear that I'll never get to sleep unless you sit and talk with me some more."

Yawning, Morgan nodded good-naturedly. He loosened his tie, and kicked off his own shoes. "There's brandy in the liquor cabinet. Would you like some?"

"Yes, please," Sonny nodded, watching him.

He poured her some into a goldfish bowl sized snifter, brought it over, and settled down beside her on the couch, propping up his stockinged feet on the coffee table.

Sonny took a sip of her brandy and sighed. "So this is what it's like to be rich. Fabulous restaurants and beautiful hotels. I could get used to this."

"No reason why you shouldn't," Morgan said. "If you take the job, you'll be doing a lot of traveling. Business is stressful enough. You need to be able to unwind in pleasant surroundings."

"But even if you can afford all this," her gesture swept the parlor, "there's so much to know." Sonny said. "About tonight's food, and the wine, for instance. How did you ever learn it all?" She shook her head, exasperated. "I feel positively unworthy to have eaten tonight. I feel like the food deserved better than my unsophisticated gut."

Morgan laughed. "I've told you before that I take great pleasure in introducing you to things. I guess it's because it was your father who taught *me* a lot about appreciating good food and wine."

"So tonight was how you usually eat?" She set her brandy down on the coffee table and sidled closer to Morgan, resting her head against his shoulder.

"God, no!" Morgan exclaimed. "This is fun, of course, but tomorrow, I'll take you to dinner at a Left Bank steak joint I like, off the Rue de la Huchette. We're talking grill smoke and sawdust on the floor. We'll sit on a bench, crammed together with the other customers—students and the like—at a communal table. The steak comes one way: served for two, or however many are in your party, with pommes frites, on a wooden plank. You help yourself to as much bread and wine as you want; the loaves are sticking up out of baskets by the front door, and the carafes are passed back and forth along the table."

"It sounds great," Sonny said.

"It *is* great. That's why I go there. *Great* is what I care about. What it *is* ain't important, as long as it's great. I can be as content with a cheeseburger as I was with tonight's *Canette de Barbarie au Cassis,* as long as it's the best of its kind."

"*Canette—*"

"*Canette de Barbarie au Cassis,*" Morgan finished for her. "It's what we ate tonight."

"Let's see," Sonny said. "That was either the lamb chops that cost so much they should have come with a sweater, or the duck smothered in hot jam, right?"

"You're lucky that it's too late for me to send you to bed without supper."

"You could *take* me to bed," Sonny said, cuddling closer.

Morgan froze.

"Morgan?" She was trailing her fingers through his hair. "Take me to bed?" she asked again, her voice very small. She moved closer, which Morgan wouldn't have thought could be possible. He felt her breasts, rising and falling with her breathing, against his arm. She began to nibble at his ear.

Damn, he was tempted. She was a beautiful woman, and he had to admit to himself that he was very much attracted to her, but her father's ghost stood between them.

Morgan slid away, turning to face her on the couch. "Sonny, you're very wonderful, but—"

"Shut up, Morgan." She stood up, looking very pale, her sensual mouth compressed into a thin, hard line. "So what if I spent a mint on this dress, and I basically threw myself at your feet, and you're looking at me like I'm dog poop. I mean, so what?"

"Sonny, I'm sorry . . ."

"Shut up! Don't apologize. I already feel enough like a fool, thank you very much."

"You're overreacting."

"*Overreacting?* You *want* overreacting, I'll *give* you overreacting," she grabbed the brandy snifter off the table and drew back her arm to hurl it. "I can't!" she grimaced. "I can't throw it, because everywhere I look in this fucking room I see a fucking antique." She put the snifter back on the table. "I bet that wouldn't have stopped Nicole Houel, right? She would have thrown the thing and not given a shit about the antiques, right? But then Nicole Houel has *class,* she has sophistication, élan; she's got *bigger tits!*"

"Sonny—"

"Not another word out of you, Morgan! If you don't want to sleep with me that's just fine—" She stalked barefooted across the carpeting to her bedroom door, then stopped, and whirled around. "No, it *isn't* fine. It stinks—" She went inside her room, slamming the door shut behind her. A second later the door slammed open. "No, *stinks* doesn't accurately express my feelings. It *sucks.*"

"Sonny, listen to me."

"It sucks *dead rats*—"

"Will you just keep quiet for one second!"

"No! Don't say anything, Morgan," she yelled. "If you say anything, if, God help you, you try to explain, I'll be forced to kill you, and that would probably affect my career path."

"Just calm down, and listen—"

"There's nothing to listen to, Morgan. I've been trying my best to get you to notice me as somebody other than Lee Thomas' daughter, and I might as well have been banging my head against a wall. I see it all, now: you prefer redheads, with funny accents and *oodles* of world-weary sophistication. If *that's* what turns you on, that's fine; that's okay. You can just forget I ever mentioned going to bed with you." She was trembling with fury, and her eyes were looking wet. "Make believe I never said a word!"

"Please calm down, Sonny—"

She pointed a shaking finger at him. "You know what I'm going to do? I'm going to drive in that publicity race, and I'm going to become a DonSport V.P., and I'm going to get so *goddamned* sophisticated it'll give you the hard-on of your life! I might even cultivate an accent, just to get you hotter, and then you just *try* and touch me! You just try it, Mister! I'll, I'll sue you for sexual harassment!"

She was on a full-tilt crying jag, now. As Morgan stared helplessly she again slammed the door shut, only to again open it. "You know what I'll do? I'll tell Artie Neal, and he'll beat you up! I might even *marry* Artie, because what do *you* care?"

Morgan desperately wanted to comfort her. He held

his arms out. "Honey, you know I feel like a father toward you—"

"Goddammit!" Sonny's shriek cut him off. "You're *not* my father!"

Her door once again slammed shut, this time for good.

9

MORGAN STARED AT Sonny's closed bedroom door. He thought he could hear her muffled sobs. A thousand thoughts were going through his mind. 1998 of them had to do with Sonny, nude, doing indescribable things to him in bed. The next to the last thought concerned Lee Thomas; specifically what Thomas might have thought about Morgan bedding his daughter. The last thought was a particularly bitter ironic one: all along he had been obsessed with the idea that Sonny had betrayed him. It had never occurred to him, until just this moment, that *he* was the one doing both professional and emotional damage to *her*.

He stood there, continuing to stare at the closed door, feeling awful, and appalled at his own helplessness. Morgan's moral no-win situation was so laughably inane. It was a classic: Sonny had what amounted to a schoolgirl crush on him, and no matter what he did about it, it would cause her pain. Nonetheless it didn't make him any less sexually aroused at the thought of making love to her. He knew he wasn't supposed to think with his cock, but he couldn't help himself. He was trying to stay high-minded, but what kept intruding was the image of Sonny in his arms; holding her, kissing her, loving her—

Fuck it, the point was, it wasn't going to happen at all.

He went into his bedroom. It was midnight, and he

122

was physically tired, but his mind was racing a mile a minute. He knew that there was no chance of sleep.

He paced the room, thinking about what Sonny had said: that she intended to drive in the Le Mans publicity race, provided he could make it happen, of course. Morgan knew that she'd made her decision in the white heat of anger, but he also knew enough about Sonny to know that she wouldn't dream of backing down once she said she would do something. He'd also believed her when she'd said that she wanted to take the management position at DonSport just to show him what she could do, even if it meant being ostracized from racing. Morgan knew that she really did want the job, but he couldn't duck the realization that he was tricking her into doing something for him that he couldn't do himself; he was tricking her into saving his ass.

Which was what he'd forced her father to do . . .

It was all wrong; damningly wrong. All along Morgan had intended to absolve himself of the sin he'd committed, and now here he was about to repeat that sin all over again, because he didn't know what else to do.

His bed looked inviting, but he knew himself too well. The last thing he wanted to do was be stretched out on his bed in the dark, staring wide-eyed into the blackness and brooding over his fucked-up past, worse present, and, seemingly, just as dismal future.

He began to undress, figuring to change into casual clothes and go out for a walk. As he stepped out of his trousers his hard cock sprang through the fly slit of his Jockey shorts.

All he had to do was step out of his room and walk across the parlor. He'd knock on her door, murmur some nonsense to placate her hurt feelings, and then enfold her soft sweetness in his arms . . .

No way. He was weak, and bad, but he wasn't evil.

He put on a pair of jeans, a turtleneck sweater, and

Nikes. He grabbed his trenchcoat and headed for the bedroom door. With his hand on the knob, he paused. He went back into the room, sat down on the edge of his bed and picked up the bedside telephone. He was going out, all right, but not for any damned walk. He knew just where he intended to go, and he figured he might as well call Nicole Houel first, to make sure that she wanted the company.

He stepped out of his bedroom with his trenchcoat on. As soon as he'd hung up on Nicole he'd called downstairs to the front desk, to have the Bristol's doorman get him a taxi for the trip across the Seine to Nicole's Left Bank hotel.

He was halfway across the parlor when Sonny's bedroom door clicked open, and he was confronted by her very large, red-rimmed, brown eyes. Her dark hair was down around her shoulders. She was wearing a pale blue silk robe, cinched tightly around her narrow waist, but spread open at the top to reveal her low-cut, pale blue negligee. It's ivory lace neckline was held together by a big, floppy, satin bow just below where her lovely cleavage began. She looked slightly ridiculous, sort of irresistible, but why should her appearance be any less painfully contrary than Morgan's feelings about her?

"Where are you going?" she asked, her voice plaintive, hoarse from crying. She shifted her stance. The fluid silk robe's bottom half parted, and one of her long, tanned legs showed through.

Morgan's heart was breaking. He wanted to be with her, but he was going to do the right thing this time, even if everything else he did was wrong.

"Just out for a walk, honey," he gently replied.

"No you're not," she shook her head mournfully. "You're going to see *her*."

How could she know? Could she guess? A little voice inside of Morgan said that she'd been eavesdropping. Another little voice said don't be a jerk; scary as it is, accept the fact that she just *knew*. "No, really, I'm not," Morgan pretended to smile. "I'm—"

Sonny's door clicked shut.

Hell, it was just one more little white lie, Morgan told himself as he stepped out into the hotel corridor. What was one more little lie?

10

SONNY WAITED UNTIL she was sure Morgan had left the suite, and then she went out into the parlor, intending to drown her sorrows in a stiff drink. It was all so laughable that she couldn't help thinking, even as she continued to sniffle: here she was in Paris—the City of Lights, of Romance, dammit—and she was no better off than she was in her little apartment back in San Francisco. Actually, she was worse off. Back home she could at least turn on the tube for company while she sat around in her jammies mooning over Don Morgan. Here in "Gay Paree" there wasn't a goddamned thing in this hotel room to look at but these fucking antiques.

She finished the brandy that Morgan had poured for her earlier and got herself another. She took it back to the sofa, where she curled up in a fetal position and moped.

It sounded impossibly corny, but hers was a case of love at first sight. Well, maybe not at *first* sight, but she did remember how on her tenth birthday she blew out the candles on the cake while making a heartfelt wish that "Uncle Donnie" would marry her. There'd been a lot of changes in her life since then, but that wish had remained a constant.

That tenth birthday party had taken place in California. Sonny remembered the palm trees in the backyard; they made an indelible impression on Sonny and her sisters, all of whom had up to that point spent their lives in Europe. Her father had been driving for BXI, an

American-based racing syndicate, and had settled the family in Los Angeles, for the climate, and to take advantage of America's more favorable income tax situation. By then Morgan had taken over her father's old job as DeManto's chief driver. He was married to a would-be starlet, or model; Sonny couldn't remember which, nor could she remember the woman's name— just that Morgan's late wife had been blonde, and German, and that she'd died a year or so after the marriage took place. At the time, Sonny's mother had concocted some story about the woman having an incurable disease when Sonny had pestered her about the incident. Much later, Sonny learned the truth: that the poor woman had been a junkie. When Morgan's wife died, Sonny couldn't help feeling pleased because it meant that her beloved was once again available. Maybe she'd been callous, but hell, she couldn't have been more than twelve or thirteen at the time; at that age death is an inconceivably remote thing, and, anyway, her hormones had been raging.

She remembered how she used to masturbate herself to sleep most every night to the most *sizzling* fantasies, all of which featured Don Morgan. (And what did she mean, *used to* . . . Even now, whether she was diddling herself, or she was with someone, her mind inevitably resurrected her old, familiar fantasies concerning Morgan in order for her to get off.)

Sonny knocked back the last of her brandy, brooding on how it was high time that she got that whole, sticky, libidinal scene under control. It was embarrassing, to say the least, when sexual fantasies intruded on real life without their owner's consent. She remembered— *because how would she ever forget?*—that time in bed with Artie when she had lost it and actually called out Morgan's name as she climaxed. *Poor Artie:* he'd looked down at her with an expression on his face like he'd come out of a trance to find himself fucking his mother. His cock had deflated faster than a balloon in a pin factory. Even now, it was hard for her not to feel absolutely terrible—or crumble into hysterical laughter —at the thought of it . . .

Poor, poor Artie. He was really a very nice boy. He really was, Sonny thought. She decided to toast Artie with another brandy. It took her only a few seconds to get to her oddly rubbery legs, and sashay her lonely little fanny over to the liquor cabinet to pour herself another teensy-weensy drink.

"To Arthur Neal, Esquire," Sonny announced to the empty room, "any *sane* woman's dream catch: a considerate, handsome man with lots of dough and a bright future. To the man who pays attention to me and who thinks of me as the woman I truly am. To the man who will doubtless ask me to marry him."

She waved the sloshing brandy snifter in the direction of the disapproving military officers glaring at her from the paintings in the room. What had Morgan said about them? About those incredibly vibrant still lifes?

"I'm going to *know* stuff like who the hell painted you," she vowed to the portraits, collapsing onto the sofa while cradling and steadying her drink because it wouldn't do to get the fucking antiques wet. She'd meant it when she told Morgan that she was going to drive in his silly race, and take the job he was offering her, and become so drop-dead chic that Morgan would positively pine away for her. But she hadn't meant it when she said that she was going to marry Arthur Neal. That had just been bluster born of some misguided hope on her part that Morgan would immediately fall to his knees and beg her to reconsider, to marry *him*.

"Fat chance," Sonny muttered into the brandy snifter. It sounded funny; muffled kind of; like when you talked through a cardboard toilet paper tube, not that she did that a lot, of course, but every once and a while, while changing the roll, she'd go 'wooo-wooo' through the empty tube, and why was the room spinning so? You'd think a zillion dollar hotel like the Bristol could keep their fucking rooms from spinning.

She gingerly set the brandy snifter down on the

coffee table and stretched out on the sofa. She tried closing her eyes, but that just made the room whirl faster. Better to keep them open, she decided, and think pleasing thoughts to combat the nauseating dizziness.

"Think about driving," she said out loud. *"Yeahhh, driving—"*

She never got dizzy when she drove. She was always in control, incapable of losing it when she was behind the wheel. She was too good. She was the best. Maybe not the best in the world, but she was sure the fucking best of her peers.

She'd always been a track brat, hanging out around the garages, and pits and paddocks as much as her parents would let her. She vividly remembered how she would sit in her daddy's lap as he took his DeManto Formula One on test loops. Once they'd settled in California, during the off-season, her daddy regularly took her to drive go-karts. As soon as she was old enough to get her driver's license she started out driving a beat-up Triumph TR3 in a few road races— they were moré like rallies, really—under the auspices of the SCCA. The Sports Car Club of America was the only major racing organization that would tolerate a woman driving. Hell, NASCAR and most of the others wouldn't even let a woman in the pits, never mind sit in a driver's seat.

She'd been good, right from the start, and had gotten steadily better with practice. She moved into Formula Vee, and it wasn't long before she had a shelf full of trophies. She used to gaze at them, wishing that her father could have seen them, but, of course, he'd been dead a whole lot of years by then.

She'd only gotten better and better as the years passed. It was like her driving potential was limitless, like there was no way she could ever peak. Even today she believed that the only thing that could stop her from going all the way, from becoming the very best, was the fact that she was a woman. Hell, right now she could drive the balls clean off any of the DonSport test drivers.

Marty Robbins knew that.

Morgan knew it, too.

She laughed out loud.

Maybe she could even drive the balls off Morgan. She couldn't have outdriven him when he was in his prime, of course. Sonny had been just a kid, but she'd never forget just how awesome a driver Morgan had been during his prime.

She hadn't actually seen very much of Morgan, except at races, during that period. He was living in London in those days, and anyway, Morgan and her father had had some kind of falling out; over what, she never knew, but she did remember how concerned and worried her father had been about Morgan. She remembered the hushed, whispered conversations about him between her father and mother, conversations that would always abruptly end when she or her sisters entered the room.

By inadvertently eavesdropping on one of her father's telephone conversations she'd learned that DeManto had fired Morgan due to his drinking. She'd been totally crushed by the news. She'd moped about, despondent, liable to break into tears at any instant, and had totally frustrated her parents by refusing to tell them what was bothering her so. It was only when her father managed to get Morgan to stop drowning his sorrows over the loss of his wife in booze, and then gave him a job as a relief driver, that Sonny was able to snap out of what her mother called her "pre-pubescent blues." Her father's ride was still with BXI, and he was doing well that year, which was lucky for Morgan, because the management at BXI had wanted nothing to do with a "has-been" like Don Morgan. Sonny proudly recalled how her father had gone out on a limb, putting his own ride on the line, to be able to hire Morgan. For a while it looked like BXI was going to call his bluff, but they'd backed down. Once Morgan was back under her father's wing he seemed to regain a little of his old magic. There's no telling what would have happened; how far the reunited team of Thomas and Morgan might have gone—

If Le Mans hadn't happened.

When Sonny and her sisters were toddlers the whole family accompanied Lee Thomas on his tours, but once they'd settled in California the family stayed put when her father went off to drive, so as not to disrupt the kids' school year. That's how it was when her father, with Morgan as his relief driver, went to Le Mans to drive for BXI. Sonny had been all alone in the basement family room, watching the race on the old twenty-seven inch Zenith that had been bumped from its position in the living room by a new RCA. Morgan had just finished his driving stint, and now Sonny's father was taking over. Her mother and sisters were watching upstairs in the living room, but Sonny, with a little girl's typical self-consciousness, liked to watch her father's races by herself, so that she didn't have to feel silly in front of the others as she pretended to drive along with him. That's what she was doing—sitting on the old Lazy-Boy recliner with its torn, red, Naugahyde patched with silver duct tape, going *varoom-varoom* and pretending to do heel and toe work—when she saw her father's pine green BXI Formula One come out from under the Dunlop bridge and *lose it*.

The car careened off a guard rail, throwing sparks like an acetylene torch. By then Sonny's scream was melding with those of her mother and sisters upstairs. She stared as her father's car flipped onto its side and then began cartwheeling end over end, before coming to rest in a blossom of orange flame and oily gray smoke.

At her daddy's funeral, everyone thought that Morgan would show up drunk, but he didn't. He was stone-cold sober that day, and, likely, sober ever since.

Sonny, despite her own, utter despair over the loss of her father, could remember how forlorn and stricken

Morgan had been on that awful day. He'd kept repeating that it should have been him. Sonny had gone over to him, and shyly taken his hand. Morgan had reached down to stroke her hair . . .

Sonny sat up on the sofa. She was no longer drunk. She was no longer angry at Morgan. She was no longer much of anything.

She wished like hell that she could go for a drive.

Her mother had been furious when, at seventeen, Sonny had announced her intention of following as far as possible in her father's footsteps. DonSport had been flourishing by then, and Morgan's checks were paying her sisters' college tuition. Her mother had pleaded with her to be like her sisters, to go to college. She could always drive for a hobby, her mother had said.

Sonny wasn't interested in remaining an amateur. If anybody had asked her, she would have responded, arrogantly but truthfully, that she was *too good* to be an amateur. Still, there was another, far more imperative motive behind her ambitions: when she was driving, she felt as if she were communing with her father. He'd died long before she was old enough to get behind the wheel of anything but a go-kart, of course, but from the very beginning, when as a little girl she'd confessed her desire to race, he hadn't laughed, but had very seriously told her that she was capable of accomplishing anything she set out to do.

Now, when she was driving on a track, Lee Thomas was with her in the car. That's what made her love driving so much. That's what made her so good. It was one part like she was a little girl again, sitting on her father's lap behind the wheel; one part that she had her father beside her as her copilot. Lately, driving fast on a track, competing with and *beating* the other drivers, seemed to be the only thing that could get her head right, put things back into proper perspective.

That was all going to change, of course. Once she pulled this stunt of masquerading as Morgan at Le

Mans, no racing organization would ever again recognize her. The taboo she was about to break was just way too large . . .

"But that's okay," Sonny told the silent portraits. "If my competition days are going to end, I want it to happen at Le Mans. This is the only way a woman could drive there, and I want to beat that fucking circuit."

Sonny grinned fiercely at the thought. Le Mans had claimed the father, but very soon now, the *daughter* was going to *own* Le Mans. It hadn't occurred to her during dinner with Morgan, but now that she'd thought it through she had not the slightest doubt that she would win that race. As her father had told her, there wasn't anything that Sonny Thomas couldn't do.

Well, there *was* one thing, maybe: make Morgan fall in love with her.

But as far as Morgan was concerned, she might as well still be ten years old, blowing out the candles on her birthday cake, making a wish that evidently could never come true.

11

MORGAN'S CABDRIVER WAS Arabic, and could have had a kamakazi-short but brilliant career in Formula One Grand Prix. He drove like a maniac, a real whammer-jammer hot-foot, cursing at the traffic in his native tongue, and taking every signal, sign, or pedestrian in his path as a personal affront not to be endured.

The cabbie did get Morgan to his destination in fifteen minutes, without ever once touching the brake pedal of his rumple-fendered, rain-slicker yellow Peugeot. There was only one good thing—besides its brevity—about the savage ride: it served to take Morgan's mind off of Sonny . . . at least, for a little while.

Morgan knew and liked the Hôtel du Carrousel. He used to stay here years ago, before he could afford the Bristol. The small, well-kept hotel—it took its name from the nearby Pont du Carrousel—was more like a luxurious inn, really, but it occupied one of the most fabulous chunks of real estate in Paris: a tree shaded, Left Bank quay that afforded most of its thirty or so rooms a view of the Louvre, directly across the narrow Seine.

The lights were dimmed over the hotel's modest entrance, but the concierge was on duty at the front desk, just by the small bar and adjoining sitting room, both of which were dark for the night. Morgan waited as the old fellow in his worn cardigan took his time looking up Nicole's room number, and then phoning up to assure himself she was receiving visitors.

The concierge hung up the telephone and despondently waved Morgan on. He went up in a phone booth–sized open grillwork elevator that took so long to drone and wheeze its way up the three floors that Morgan could have shimmied up the damned cable faster. Nicole answered the door at his first knock. She hauled him inside, took the cigarette from out of the corner of her mouth, kissed him passionately, and then stuck the Pall Mall back between her lips.

"I am so glad you're here," she said in her languorous, French-tinged English. "I was just thinking about you when you called. I was thinking how nice it would be tonight if you were to come over."

Her unruly red mane had been loosely bundled into a ponytail. She had a pencil tucked behind her ear. She wasn't wearing makeup, but she didn't need any. Her peachy, lightly freckled complexion was flawless, her pouting lips were deliciously pink, and her emerald eyes glittered like precious stones. She was wearing a gray cotton tank top and matching jockey shorts; it was that men's locker room inspired stuff they were lately hard-selling the ladies. Call him old-fashioned, but Morgan still preferred his sex objects in lace and satin. Nicole's tank top was losing the push-pull battle to contain her full breasts, and when she turned to lead him into the room, Morgan noticed that the backside of her briefs had bunched up between the cheeks of her round, pale bottom. It was a view that was even more breathtaking than the marble-like curves of the Louvre looming outside the room's lace curtained, floor-to-ceiling windows, but gray Jockey shorts were still gray Jockey shorts. It occurred to Morgan that Sonny was a woman who could look deliciously sexy in such tomboy drag, and then it occurred to Morgan to stop thinking about Sonny.

Nicole's smallish room was adequately furnished in that perfectly proper but nondescript manner that is the French bourgeoisie's answer to Holiday Inn. The room was also incredibly messy. The desk was littered with all the signs of a high tech literary work in progress: a portable laptop computer and a modem shared space with yellow legal pads, manila folders, her little tape recorder, and a half-filled bottle of cognac and a glass. Ashtrays overflowing with butts were everywhere, as were crumbled up balls of canary yellow paper. On the other side of the massive armoire that served as the room's closet was a door leading to a small, white tiled bathroom. Nicole had a pastel confetti of washed out panties hanging, or spread to dry, on every possible porcelain or chromed surface, including the bidet.

"Why are you in a hotel? When we met, I seem to remember you saying that you lived in Paris," Morgan commented.

"I didn't say that." She padded over to the unmade, double bed and flopped down, in a cross-legged position. "I only said that I met Niles in Paris."

"Oh. Well, you have a good memory."

"It is necessary for a journalist," she nodded intently.

"Oh." Morgan waited, and when it was evident she was prepared to let him wait a long time, he asked, "So, where *do* you live?"

"Here, there, everywhere."

"Yeah, that was a nice Beatles tune, but the question was where do you live?"

She made a big production out of sighing and looking weary. "Often, I think I live out of a suitcase. You see, I travel almost constantly."

"You just don't want to tell me where you live, do you?"

"Does it matter so much?"

"Okay," Morgan surrendered. "Who am I to call anyone eccentric?" He looked around at the mess. "My next question is did you recently suffer a burglary, or do you always live like this?"

She took one last puff of her smoke, then dropped it into the dregs of the coffee cup on the night table; it sizzled out with what sounded like a little hiss of amused disdain. "When I work, I can't be bothered with keeping neat." She looked down at herself. "And I find that too many layers of clothing constrict my thoughts." She winked at him as she pulled at the tank top, stretching it down beneath her tits, to display her swelling nipples. They looked rouged, but Morgan knew that they were all natural, with no artificial coloring or flavoring added. "Do you approve of my clothing?" she asked.

"I'd like to peel you out of that tomboy stuff, because your type doesn't belong in it."

She laughed. "Tell me more about 'my type'."

"Your type needs to be dressed in the seamed nylons and black garter belt your wicked self was born to wear."

"Well," Nicole licked her lips. "it's still early."

Morgan sat down beside her on the bed and began to kiss her. He began to stroke her soft thigh. Nicole slid her hands up beneath his turtleneck sweater and began playing with his nipples.

"Are you going to get undressed?" she asked, breathless, "Or will you fuck me in your trenchcoat and sneakers?"

"Yes, I think so. As this is Paris, the trenchcoat will be in memory of Humphrey Bogart."

"And the sneakers?" Nicole asked. She'd unzipped his jeans, and her lithe and busy journalist's fingers had begun touchtyping along his cock.

"The sneakers are in honor of Speedy Gonzales."

She gave him a little squeeze. "You'd better *not* be."

He wasn't.

He lost the trenchcoat and the sneakers in the tussle, as well as the rest of his clothes, but Nicole's Little League skivvies didn't last too long, either. He made sure Nicole enjoyed herself, and he had a good, if not fantastic, time. It was kind of like the sexual equivalent of taking a leak after a long, bumpy car ride. It was basically a relief. At some point Nicole, writhing, started in with her hissed Gallic imprecations and guttural squallings. Morgan stayed quiet, involved in his work, although he did curse softly when he came. It wasn't due to sensation, or passion, but because at that moment he found himself flashing on Sonny, all alone in her bed in that ridiculous, heartrendingly lovely, floppy bow tied negligee—a marvelous, neglected present he could never unwrap.

Morgan dozed off, and then awoke to Nicole burrowing under the covers, her mouth finding him. He remained in his blissful half-asleep state, content to let her do most of the work. When she had him ready, she swung around to straddle him, and it was very nice to fall back asleep beneath her moist warmth.

They were both awakened by the gurgling rumble of the first of the morning's tour boats cruising past on the Seine, just a few yards beyond the room's big windows. They took a shower together. It was a tight squeeze into the shower stall, but they managed it.

"I think this is the outfit I like you in best," Morgan told her, gliding the soap along her breasts and the curve of her belly, and then gently kneading a creamy lather into the ruddy thatch between her thighs. "Just dripping wet."

"Then keep me that way," Nicole laughed, rubbing her nipples against his chest, taking the soap from him and rubbing it in circles down his back and along the crack of his ass. He fucked her one last time, the two of them standing up in the warm, cascading shower spray; he kept at her until she yelped.

After they were dried and dressed, they left the hotel and walked along the Quay Voltaire, squinting in the molten sunlight glinting on the river, until they found a cafe. They took a small table away from the sleepy-eyed regulars who were congregated around the espresso machine, and ordered café au lait and croissants, hot from the baker's oven, with sweet butter and orange marmalade.

"I understand you and Niles have come to a business agreement," Nicole said, after they'd been served.

Morgan nodded. "Pretty much, although there are still some financial details to be worked out."

"Niles definitely has his heart set on the race at Le Mans," Nicole said. "That, and having those cars tour your country."

"*That* part won't be a problem. Niles has agreed to flat-out buy the cars if the manufacturers won't lend them. My main concern is getting the manufacturers to agree to participate in the race, in the first place."

"Do you think you will succeed?" she asked.

"I'd better, if I want this deal to go through. Niles was very clear about that."

"Niles *can* be intractable when he has his heart set on something," Nicole agreed. She took a sip of her coffee. "Do you suppose it was his stubborness that caused him to lose so much money gambling?"

Morgan smiled. "You've mentioned that before, and I've told you before that I didn't know anything about that. I thought you had a great memory?"

"Oh, yes, that's right, you said you didn't care for Niles. Quite a coincidence that you and he are now involved in this major business deal." She lit a cigarette, and waved out the match.

"Do you?" Morgan challenged. "Like Niles, I mean."

"Why, are you jealous?" She smiled through the veil of cigarette smoke.

"Should I be?"

"It depends." She busied herself shaping her cigarette's ash against the edge of the ashtray. When she looked up her green eyes tracked him like guns. "How much do you want?"

Morgan grinned. "Niles told me you were quite agreeable to the idea of working closely with me." When she nodded, he added, "That could mean very long days—"

"And nights." The tip of her pink tongue darted out at him. "We must not forget the long, long nights."

"I think we both want the same thing," Morgan said.

"We will see."

"I was surprised when Niles said you'd volunteered for the job as press liaison," Morgan said. "I would have thought that you were far too busy for that sort of job."

"Well, fortunately, I am busy," Nicole said. "But I told you yesterday how much I love fast cars and fast men. When Niles suggested the job to me, I knew I wanted to do it. I figure to squeeze in some extra hours of writing to meet my other deadlines. As a matter of fact, I was working on a story last night, which is why you caught me in."

"Lucky me," Morgan said.

"Lucky us."

"I saw one of your stories on art theft in yesterday's *Tribune*," Morgan told her.

"You mentioned that," she nodded, looking pleased. "It's a fascinating subject."

"But kind of esoteric," Morgan said. "I mean, it hardly affects a lot of people, the way, say, drug dealing does."

"Well, art thievery doesn't foster a lot of low level, violent street crime, if that's what you mean," Nicole admitted. "But it costs us, nevertheless, in insurance premiums, for instance. In Europe it is very wide-spread. Say you spent the day visiting some of the museums here in Paris. By the time you were done you would have likely looked at dozens of stolen pieces."

Morgan stared at her in disbelief. "In the straight *museums?* I mean, I *know* there are crooked galleries that fence this stolen stuff, but *respectable museums* traffic in hot art?"

"Oh, all the time! The museums and auction houses are quite as bad as the crooked galleries, Morgan. Actually, the museums and auction houses are worse than the galleries, because they are hypocrites." She laughed. "Actually, they are more like the masochists, you know? They beg for more abuse, even as they moan about their hurt."

"I don't understand," Morgan frowned. "If those institutions know the art is stolen, why do they buy it?"

"For the same reason people buy your ridiculously expensive, gaudy cars," she smiled. "Because people are greedy; they *covet;* they wish to own what others cannot. And, unlike cars, it is practically impossible to prove that objets d'art are stolen. The art world fosters conspiracy." Nicole paused to light a cigarette off of the smouldering butt of her last. "Their businesses are *so* genteel; *très discret,* yes? It would never do for the museum curator who covets a particular painting to probe too deeply into the sales history of the work. If he did, the seller would likely take his offering elsewhere. The same goes with the auction houses." She shook her head in disgust. "But when the museums and auction houses suffer a theft, they cry for the authorities to do something."

"Your article was about organized crime. How does it fit into this?"

"The mob might order some artwork stolen by freelance specialists who are paid up front for their work." She paused. "It used to be that these freelancers often made life simple for the authorities by turning around and informing on whoever had hired them."

"Yeah, I read that in your article," Morgan said.

"The police often even arranged for the freelancers to receive the reward being offered. In this sort of crime, catching those who finance the operation, and getting back the stolen property, is of the utmost importance."

"But, as you wrote, now that these pros are working for the mob, informing to the cops would not be healthy," Morgan nodded.

"The freelancers are far more afraid of the mob than they are the authorities," Nicole agreed. "Anyway, once organized crime has the stolen art, the piece can be disposed of in several ways. They can launder it by forging papers and putting it back on the market, selling it out of one of their own galleries. They can sell it to a museum, a transaction relatively easy for the mob to arrange, as here in Europe organized crime has infiltrated the boards of directors of most of these institutions. If the stolen piece was heavily insured, the mob can simply demand a ransom for its return."

"But the insurance companies don't pay, do they?"

"By demanding less than the piece is insured for, the mob makes it sound business practice for the insurance company to pay."

"But it's cutting their own throats," Morgan argued. "It's like a terrorist/hostage situation: acquiescing does nothing but encourage further crimes."

Nicole shrugged. "That's easy to say, but the reality is that a ransom is only money, and a work of art, like a hostage's life, is irreplaceable." She smiled. "And because the artwork is irreplaceable, it appreciates with time, which brings me to the final way for organized crime to deal with their booty. They can simply put it in a bank vault, and wait for the statute of limitations on the crime to run out. There are added advantages to this method: at that point the item can be legally offered for sale, which means it can command a much higher price, and, of course, as I already mentioned, the piece has likely appreciated during the time it was hidden away."

Morgan shook his head. "You sure know a lot about all of this."

"As a journalist it is my job to research my subjects thoroughly," Nicole said. "I have spent much time at Interpol headquarters, both here and in other countries, combing the files and interviewing experts. I also have some underworld contacts who will talk to me because they know I am committed to protecting my sources."

"It seems like the law can't get a handle on these art thieves," Morgan said.

"There is one way," Nicole said. "Greed is their Achilles heel. You see, it is very easy to smuggle stolen art back and forth across European borders. The criminals would be relatively safe if they were content to keep their goods here. But these days, those willing to pay the really big money are Americans, and to a lesser extent, the Japanese."

"Why America?" Morgan asked.

"In your country's southwestern and sunbelt cities there are numerous recently endowed museums hungry to line their walls with art, and very often willing to look the other way concerning where their acquisitions come from. And then there are the private collectors, the nouveaux riches who would lock away a stolen masterpiece. The fact that they cannot show it off doesn't seem to matter to them," Nicole continued. "They take satisfaction merely in the knowledge that something priceless is now their property."

"So what you're saying is like with cars, there's an American gray market for art?"

Nicole nodded. "To satisfy that market, the mob must open up their vault, bring their stolen goods out of hiding, and then figure a way to smuggle them into your country."

"And that's where the cops can get them, huh? At customs? That's interesting." He glanced at his watch.

"I'm so sorry," Nicole exclaimed. "I have been boring you."

"Not at all. It was very interesting, but . . ."

"But more than you had bargained for, yes?" She blushed. "I do apologize. I get carried away with my work."

"I hope you can get as involved in your work for me," Morgan smiled.

"Oh, I will," she smiled back. "So! What are your plans for the day?"

"I've got a few loose ends to tie up at the Salon." Morgan put some francs down on the table to settle the bill. "I leave for Italy tomorrow morning."

"Will I see you tonight?"

"I don't think so. My plane leaves very early tomorrow morning. If things go well in Italy, I'll be seeing you at Le Mans next week."

He went back to the Bristol to change clothes. When he arrived, Sonny wasn't in the suite.

He grabbed a cab to La Défense quarter, and finished up his business at the Salon. It would be continuing for several more days, so Morgan wasn't worried about the manufacturers pulling their cars out of Paris. While he was there, Morgan remained on the lookout for Sonny, but she didn't seem to be around.

Late in the afternoon he returned to the hotel. He checked her bedroom, saw evidence that she'd been there while he was gone, and felt relieved to at least know that she hadn't been kidnapped by terrorists, or something. Okay, so she was avoiding him. That was understandable. But she was going to have to come back sooner or later. Morgan would wait for her right here in the suite. She couldn't avoid him forever.

It turned out that she was able to avoid him for quite a long time. At about 8:30 Morgan gave up on her and went out to get something to eat on his own. He took the metro to the Place St. Michel, intending to follow through on his plan to go to his Left Bank steak joint. He'd been looking forward to it, but by the time he'd emerged from the metro station into the bustling student quarter, he'd lost his appetite. Anyway, it wasn't the kind of place that was any fun to go to all by yourself. He walked for a while, feeling lonesome. He reminded himself that he could always call Nicole, but he knew that it was Sonny he missed.

He eventually ended up in a despicable tourist trap of an eatery on the Boulevard Saint Germain. He picked at his food, as all around him surly waiters did their best to piss off equally unhappy looking tourists. He was so down that he didn't even feel like arguing over the fact that the waiter had incorrectly added the bill in the restaurant's favor. Morgan just paid and split. Out on the street again, he decided to walk back to the Bristol, which was a goodly hike, but he desperately wanted to kill as much time as possible. He really wanted Sonny to be in the suite when he got back.

She wasn't.

Morgan sat in the parlor waiting for her, his emotions alternating between longing and dread. What could he say to her when she did come in? She finally showed up a little after midnight, dressed in jeans, sweater, running shoes, and trenchcoat.

She saw him sitting on the sofa, and paused awkwardly in the doorway. "Oh, hi."

"Hi," Morgan said brightly. "I'm glad you're okay. I was a little worried." He was so glad to see her his heart was pounding with relief.

"Yeah, well, I took the day off, and just wandered around on my own. Hope you don't mind," she added in a basically *fuck-you* tone that Morgan chose to ignore.

"No! Not at all," Morgan said, way too heartily. "Where'd you go?" He felt like a talk show host.

"Where'd *you* go last night?" Sonny shot right back, brimming over with fury that shocked Morgan in its abruptness.

"Sonny, I don't have to answer to you," Morgan began gently.

"Right, and I don't have to answer to you," Sonny replied, deliberately, sarcastically mimicking his voice-of-reason tone.

Stalemated, they looked at each other for a moment, and then Sonny shrugged. "Well, it's late. We've got to be up early tomorrow to pack, right?"

Morgan felt like crying. "Right!" His jaw ached from the effort of maintaining his phony smile.

Sonny, expressionless, looked him over a final time. "Yeah, well, good night," she said wearily.

"Sonny—"

She shook her head, not even looking at him as she made her way to her bedroom. "Morgan, I can't change the way I feel about you, but I can sure as hell repress it, okay? That's just what I'm going to do. I'd appreciate it if you'd help me out along that line by pretending that blowout we had last night never happened, okay?"

"I *would* like to discuss what happened—"

"Morgan!" she cut him off, turning to glare at him in the doorway of her bedroom. "It never happened. *Okay?*"

He couldn't look her in the eye. "Okay," he said softly in surrender.

"Good night, Morgan." She went into her bedroom, softly clicking shut the door.

"'Night," Morgan said to the empty parlor. He got up and went into his own bedroom, feeling disgusted with himself and with the entire nasty situation they had gotten themselves into. He realized that right now they were two people a million miles apart, with little hope of ever regaining even the minimal closeness they'd shared that first night.

Well, at least knowing that Sonny was safely home was somewhat comforting, he told himself. It was what he could do for her: keep her safe and well-cared for, the way her father would have taken care of her, if Lee had lived.

It wasn't much, but it was better than nothing.

12

THE NEXT MORNING Morgan and Sonny flew Alitalia nonstop from Paris to Bologna, where Morgan had called ahead to reserve a four wheel drive Ford Scorpio from the Hertz airport outlet. It was a big car; when driving in Italy Morgan liked as much sheet metal as possible between him and everyone else on the road with a death wish in their heart and a fireball Fiat in their command. Morgan would have preferred renting a Sherman tank, but Hertz was out of them, so he figured that the well-buttressed, agile Scorpio would have to do.

They were expected at the DeManto factory complex outside Modena that evening. Morgan had wired ahead to ask Professor DeManto for an audience, which the Old Man had granted, inviting Morgan and Sonny to dinner.

Modena was just about forty kilometers from Bologna, not a very long trip so they spent the day exploring Bologna's ancient, ochre piazzas, and had a fabulous lunch at Al Pappagallo on the Piazza Mercanzia, near the town's famous twin, leaning towers. Throughout the day Morgan and Sonny had been absolutely pleasant with each other.

God, it was just horrible between them. Morgan would have much rather had even a knock down, screaming fight than this sort of strained, fake cordiality.

Sonny kept up her ice queen act all through lunch. Not even the *tagliatelle alla bolognese,* veal, and the best part of a bottle of Sangiovese de Romagna could thaw her, although it was clear that an apparently broken heart did little to affect her appetite.

The day was overcast, but mild, with the temperature in the mid-seventies. Morgan dispensed with the Scorpio's air-conditioning and slid open the sunroof for the drive to Modena. Traveling the Italian autostrada was a dream compared to driving on American interstates. It was a lot like Germany's autobahn. Morgan kept the Scorpio at a steady 100 mph clip and hardly had to use his brakes, except to pull into the right lane when the *really fast* traffic wanted to pass.

"Holy shit, we just passed a cop!" Sonny called out excitedly, above the roar of the wind and banshee howl of the Scorpio's engine. "I thought for sure you were going to get a ticket, but he never even looked twice at us!"

"DeManto, Ferarri, and Maserati all have factories around here within a few miles of each other," Morgan told her, keeping his eyes on the road. "After *ragú Bolognese,* and Lambrusca, this region owes its reputation—and its wealth—to drivers who feel the need for speed. When I used to test drive DeMantos around here, the motorcycle cops would salute me when I careened past them doing 120."

Sonny laughed. Morgan glanced at her, feeling as perturbed as a teenager out with the prom queen. Well, anyway, she was laughing. Maybe it was going to be all right between them; she seemed to be thawing, after all.

The drive took half an hour. They weren't expected at the DeManto grounds until evening, so Morgan passed the Maranello exit and drove straight through to Modena. He'd booked adjoining rooms for them at the Fini. It was luxurious, but very Italian high tech, which was not really to Morgan's taste, but it had secure parking for the Scorpio, and it was located on the Via Emilia Est, just outside the center of the town, which meant less hassle fighting traffic to get back onto the autostrada for the drive to the DeManto complex. Anyway, they'd only be staying the night.

They dumped their luggage, and the car, and walked the half mile to the old quarter. They said little as they strolled the broad, tree lined Avenue Garibaldi bordered by public gardens, and then poked around the town's charming arcaded squares, and the cool, somber interior of its Cathedral. Morgan tried to absorb himself in the sights, but he just wasn't in the mood to gaze appreciatively at any more sunlit piazzas, crumbling palazzos, or leaning towers; to let his heart be warmed by the flocks of short-panted schoolboys or the theatrical antics of the aproned waiters, like contestants in a Chef Boy-ar-dee look-alike contest.

What Morgan was in the mood for was to shake Sonny out of her funk and in that way lose his own. Whatever truce she'd momentarily declared between them had evidently ended with their drive. Sonny was once again as cold as the marble friezes ornamenting the Cathedral's entrances, and Morgan was like Marley's ghost, dragged down and tormented by the heavy chains of his own inability to make things all right between them once again.

On the other hand, her melodramatic sulkiness was also beginning to piss Morgan off. Why the fuck couldn't they just be friends again? He knew what she was doing: she was playing hard to get, the oldest trick in the book—*so why the fuck was it working?* And wasn't the way Sonny was acting precisely the behavior he'd wanted from her, to relate to him in a professional, and businesslike manner? If not, what *did* he want?

How about the world? How about to have his cake and eat it, too?

"How about an espresso?" he asked Sonny, who nodded without looking at him.

They had it in a sidewalk cafe near the massive Ducal Palace, and then decided to return to the hotel to rest. The entire walk back passed in the same, uneasy silence. By the time they'd reached the hotel Morgan couldn't wait to be away from Sonny. Once he was in his own room he felt unaccountably lost and alone. He had this almost irresistible urge to go knock on Sonny's door and ask her to go to bed with him, just to break the glacier that had frozen into place between them.

Instead he undressed, took a shower, and stretched out on his bed. It was the traveling that was screwing up their previously perfect, platonic relationship, he decided; being thrown together in exotic locales was wreaking havoc with their senses of decorum, making them forget who they were and what their relationship had to be. What they needed was for this goddamned trip to be over. Once they were back in San Francisco, and once Sonny was back with Arthur Neal to take the edge off, they could resume their friendship, and mentor/protege relationship.

Yeah, what they needed (Fuck it, what *he* needed; it was painfully, obvious that Sonny had *her* emotions under control) was to be physically apart. What he needed was to escape from her magic.

Because he was falling in love with her. Despite the difference in their ages, and despite her father's hovering ghost, despite all the lies and shit from the past, Morgan was falling in love with Sonny Thomas. And there wasn't a damned thing he could do about it.

At quarter past seven Morgan and Sonny left the hotel to drive out to the DeManto complex. They took the autostrada back towards Bologna for a couple of kilometers, and then turned off onto a side road for a ten kilometer stretch. After all these years it felt very strange to Morgan to be driving these familiar old roads, to that familiar destination, especially with Sonny Thomas by his side. He'd driven these roads so many times with her father in the passenger's seat (off the track, Lee had always been content to let others do the driving).

To add to the kaleidoscopic déjà vu, Sonny was again wearing that perfume that Ilsa used to favor. The scent was filling the Scorpio's passenger compartment.

"What is the name of that perfume?" Morgan asked.

Sonny twisted around in her seat to grin at him. "Do you like it?"

"Very much."

"I thought you'd never notice. I've been wearing it for ages. It's called Vengeance."

Morgan broke up.

"What's so funny?" Sonny demanded.

"Nothing, everything," he sighed when he'd managed to stop laughing.

"Morgan," she began shyly. "About the way I've been acting . . ."

"I don't want to talk about it now," he gently cut her off. "This meeting with DeManto is crucial; I just want to think about that for the time being, okay?"

"Okay. I understand. We can talk about it later. Just know that I'm sorry for the childish way I've been acting."

"And you just remember what I told you," Morgan said. "You can't run out of chances with me."

He took his eyes off the road long enough to give her an appreciative glance. He'd asked her to dress elegantly and she'd followed through: she was wearing a knee length, slim, red satin skirt, and a black, cardigan cashmere sweater with padded shoulders, cinched tightly around her narrow waist by a wide, black leather belt. Her stockings were gray. She was wearing plain black pumps. Her dark hair was pulled tight, and sleekly twisted into a dancer's chignon. Her only jewelry was a pair of chunky, onyx and silver earrings.

Morgan was wearing a staid, charcoal gray, double-breasted wool suit and a pair of glove leather, dove gray loafers. His Turnbull & Asser shirt carried a wide, gray stripe. His hose were mauve, the exact hue of his tie's regimental striping of mauve and indigo blue. The tie was a stab at hometown civic pride: He had no idea what regiment sported mauve and indigo blue for its colors, but he figured it was a good bet they were based somewhere around San Francisco.

Professor DeManto, of course, would be in black-tie, even for this most intimate of dinners. For a man who'd made his fortune building fire-engine red, jet fighter sports cars, the Old Man had quite funereal tastes concerning matters of personal style.

Morgan slowed the Scorpio, clicking on its high beams to search out the signpost for the private road that led to the DeManto complex. He saw it: a five foot high post topped by a circular marker about the size of a frisbee. It was painted yellow, and upon it in black, was the DeManto marque of a prancing unicorn.

Morgan turned onto the steeply inclined, loosely packed, graveled surface, dropping the car into low gear, grateful to have four wheel drive traction. The Scorpio was as sure-footed as a mountain goat, but Morgan nevertheless took it slow. It'd been a long time since he'd driven this serpentine, climbing road, and a fog had begun to set in, creating swirling wraiths that wrapped around the dark tree trunks along both sides of the twisty, high banked trail.

But foggy apparitions escorting them to Professor DeManto were appropriate, Morgan thought. There were a lot of ghosts out tonight.

After a few minutes they drove through a pair of wrought iron gates, and followed the gravel road past the workshops and garage complexes in front of which a number of DeManto vehicles sat still and silent, like guardian beasts at bay. They drove on. The road led up a hill, then to the circular driveway of the main house.

"Holy shit," Sonny murmured as she gazed at the big stone house covered with ivy and surrounded by gardens, its casement windows glowing lemon-yellow, its fog-wisped turrets starkly thrust into the night sky. As they walked to the front door, Sonny said, "It's beautiful, in a monstrous sort of way." She shook her head. "I can't decide whether its a dream mansion or a haunted house."

A short, white-haired butler in a cutaway coat let them into the marble and mahogany foyer and took their coats. The servant didn't look familiar to Morgan, but then he hadn't been here in a lot of years.

"Donaldo, how good to see you—"

Fabiano Manfredi, a middle-aged man in a dark business suit with thinning hair combed straight back and a handlebar moustache, came hurrying down the sweeping staircase to greet them. Morgan had met Manfredi some years ago at a Salon, just after the man had left a rival manufacturer to become one of the Professor's proteges.

Morgan shook hands with Manfredi, and then introduced him to Sonny.

"I never had the pleasure of meeting your father, *signorina*," Mandfredi said, bowing from the waist, "but I have heard that his great talent lives on in you."

"Gee . . ." Sonny stared at him as he kissed her hand. She nodded sagely at Morgan, lifting her eyebrow as if to say, *a girl could get used to this*.

"To know that such a lovely woman waits to skillfully put my mounts to the test inspires me to new heights of automotive genuis," Mandfredi gallantly murmured.

Sonny said, "Oohhhh . . ." and beamed.

"Way to go Fabi, baby," Morgan dryly acknowledged. "So where's the Old Man?"

"Waiting for us. We'll be dining in his study," Manfredi replied. "I'll be joining you this evening, in order to act as the *Professore's* intrepreter."

"We're eating in his study?" Morgan frowned. "Not in the main dining room? That doesn't sound like the prim and proper Professor I remember."

153

Manfredi shook his head. "Donaldo, prepare yourself. He is not as you remember him. He has a cancer, you see . . ."

"I'm very sorry to hear that," Morgan said, and he meant it. He and the Old Man had had a love/hate relationship, with the emphasis on the latter these last few years, but Professor DeManto was one of the greats of automotive history. To contemplate his demise was to contemplate a diminished world.

"It seems that he has been ill for quite some time, but managed to keep his suffering from everyone," Manfredi continued. "This past year, however, it has been very bad for the *Professore*. He has confined himself to his study and his bedroom. He has not been out-of-doors for a very long time. He has taken no interest in the day-to-day affairs of the business for even longer. He just sits, sifting through his momentos, murmuring to himself." Manfredi paused. "You are his first visitors in many months."

"Doesn't he have any family?" Sonny asked.

"The Old Man's clan was wiped out during the Second World War," Morgan explained. "He never married."

"But his magnificent automobiles are his children," Manfredi proudly added. "Since he has turned all other well-wishers away, I was quite surprised when he consented to see you, Don, and, of course, the *signorina*." He graciously nodded to Sonny. "And I was even further astounded when he insisted that you come for dinner."

"Well, he knew we wished to discuss business," Morgan said.

Manfredi made a dour face. "I'm not sure that would be wise, Donaldo. The *Professore* is very weak, and his attention wanders. Perhaps you should restrict your conversation tonight to lighter subjects. Later, you can discuss your business with me."

"I prefer to have the Professor hear me out, and then speak for himself. Thanks, anyway, Fabi."

Manfredi shrugged philosophically, and then offered a smile that Morgan sensed was forced. "Perhaps your visit will mark a turnabout in his condition," Manfredi said. "Perhaps we can hope for an improvement in his health, even if it can be only temporary."

"I sincerely hope that will be so," Morgan said.

"Well," Manfredi said briskly, gesturing towards the staircase. "We mustn't keep him waiting. Please, you will follow me."

Upstairs, they walked along what seemed an endless, dimly lit, hallway, carpeted in burgundy wool. Sonny, wide-eyed, hung back a bit. She clutched at Morgan's sleeve to whisper, "This is kind of spooky."

Morgan knew what she meant: the decor was straight out of *Abbot and Costello Meet the Wolf-Man*. Besides the maze of hallways leading to God-knows-where, there were suits of armor guarding doorways, and ornately-framed oil portraits faded to the color of weak tea, with eyes that seemed to follow you around. The only thing missing was one of those bookcases you leaned on, and then it revolved to let you into the laboratory. Who knew? The Old Man probably had one of those, as well.

Manfredi knocked once upon the the study's closed door and opened it. Morgan allowed Sonny to precede him and then went in. He looked around, wondering where Professor DeManto was.

The large, shadowy, book-lined study had in its center a rectangular table covered in snowy linen. It was candle-lit, and set for four with china, silver, and crystal, but surrounding the table were only three straight-backed dining chairs. Except for that table, clearly there temporarily for this evening, the room was exactly as Morgan had remembered it: still the same somber earth tones of lustrous leather and waxed wood; the same fire perpetually crackling in that slate hearth; the same, scale-model, DeManto prototypes resting on the mantel, between the same pair of brass lamps with green glass shades. And there, beneath the heavily curtained windows, was that same sideboard laden with the many trophies garnered during the Old Man's illustrious career.

Morgan noticed Sonny staring at the treasure cache of burnished gold and ornate silver cups, glittering in the candlelight.

"Some of those were won by your father," he told her.

"And some were won by you," she whispered back, so that only Morgan could hear her. She looked up at him, her brown eyes large and somber, and squeezed Morgan's hand.

Morgan heard a metallic squeak and a rustle of cloth. From out of a dark corner, like a wolf from out of its lair, came the Old Man.

The Professor was in black tie, all right, but he was also in a wheelchair. *It's been a long time since I've seen him,* Morgan reminded himself. *It sometimes feels like it's been a lifetime and a half. He was old back then. God only knows how old he is now.*

If the study looked exactly the same, the Old Man had changed a great deal; as Fabiano Manfredi had said, the change had been for the worse. It wasn't just the wheelchair. The Old Man had always been gaunt, but now he looked skeletal, and he'd lost inches of height. His gleaming white curls were gone, revealing a mottled, almost simian skull, wreathed with coarse gray fuzz. His skin had taken on the dreary yellow tint of nicotine-stained meerschaum, and his face was a mass of wrinkles. Only the Professor's eyes seemed to have remained the same. They were still clear, black, and glittering.

Then Morgan looked closer, and realized that the Professor's eyes had changed, after all. They were now as hard as stone and just as lifeless.

Something awful had happened to this man, Morgan realized, something that went beyond physical illness. What it had been, he didn't know; only that the Professor had once been passionate and in love with life and his work. This shriveled man ludicrously trussed up in a tuxedo and peering at them from a wheelchair had the cold-blooded, expressionless eyes of a reptile.

Manfredi hurried around behind the wheelchair to push it towards Morgan and Sonny. Professor DeManto held out his gnarled, palsied hand, which Morgan gently took. It felt like ice.

DeManto craned his neck to speak to Manfredi in Italian. The Old Man's melodious whisper had turned into a harsh rasp.

Manfredi nodded in response to the torrent of Italian. "The *Professore* welcomes you, Morgan, and especially you, *signorina*. He says that it has been many years since a Thomas has graced these grounds, and DeManto has been the poorer because of it. Due to his frail health, he begs you two young people to indulge an old man for whom the evening must of necessity be brief. Please to go directly to the table."

Talk about spa cuisine. As they took their places around the table a butler appeared at the doorway with a trolley laden with shallow bowls of clear chicken consommé. The broth was followed by plain, steamed filet of sole, accompanied by a small garni of equally plain, equally steamed vegetables. The beverage was mineral water.

"I'm glad we had a big lunch," Sonny whispered to Morgan as she contemplated the lean pickings.

Morgan understood perfectly: the Old Man had never in his life had a thought for anyone else. If this was what Erberto DeManto had to eat and drink for his health, then this is what everyone would eat and drink. Morgan supposed that an egocentric mindset went along with being a genius; and nobody had ever made the claim that geniuses were easy to be around.

Morgan ate as little of the wretched food as he could without offending his host. He waited impatiently as the Old Man dawdled over his own meal. He was amused to see Sonny polishing off every morsel of food on her plate. The kid had an appetite like a horse.

Right now, Morgan's stomach was too fluttery for him to eat anything—even if something appetizing *had* been presented.

The fact that DeManto was ill did not bode well for Morgan's cause. It would take energy on DeManto's behalf to set the wheels in motion for Morgan's publicity race at Le Mans. It would cause the Old Man aggravation with his United States dealership network to agree to supply DonSport with enough cars to go nationwide. Sick old men were low on energy, and the last thing they wanted was more aggravation than their bodies were already giving them.

At last the Professor set down his fork. He'd eaten even less than Morgan had. He said something in his sawtoothed Italian to Manfredi, who, in turn, repeated the English translation to Morgan and Sonny. "The *Professore* understands that you have graced him with your visit in order to discuss a business proposition with him?"

Morgan nodded to DeManto, who was intently watching him, and launched into his pitch: the details of Nile Kingman's proposal, the idea for the publicity race, and participating cars' subsequent tour of the United States—the whole nine yards. Throughout his explanation, Morgan had to periodically wait for Mandfredi to translate passages into Italian. Morgan knew a little more Italian than he let on; from his limited knowledge he could tell that the Professor's protege disapproved of his proposal and was putting the worst possible face on the deal. There was nothing Morgan could do but hope that the Professor, though physically weak, still had a strong enough mind to hear between the lines of what his interpreter was saying.

". . . And so, I'm here to respectfully ask the *Professore* to give me his blessings on this endeavor," Morgan concluded, "to supply my expanded dealership with his fine automobiles to sell, to honor me by his marque's participation in the race, and to use his great influence to persuade others to participate."

Manfredi was frowning. "What you're asking goes against all traditional methods of doing business."

"You develop a talent for telepathy I don't know about, Fabi?" Morgan asked coldly, "Or are you advancing your own opinion?"

"I am advancing a sound business opinion," Manfredi snapped.

Morgan caught Sonny's warning glance. "Watch it, Champ," she said quietly. "You can get *yourself* KO'd trying too hard to deliver a knockout punch."

Morgan chuckled—and in the process regained his cool. "Fabiano, forgive me for raising my voice to you. But we happen to be talking about the Professor's business, not *yours.*"

Manfredi opened his mouth to reply, but the *Professore* beat him to it. It seemed to take all of his energy to speak. By the time he'd finished, he was gasping for breath, and Manfredi was staring at him in doubt. DeManto, breathing hard, pounded his fist against his chair's armrest and then savagely gestured at Morgan.

"The *Professore* has not ruled out your requests," Manfredi reluctantly began, "but he wishes to know how you could protect his American market interests if his efforts on your behalf cost him the good will of his existing dealers?"

"If necessary, DonSport America would be prepared to represent the entire DeManto line," Morgan told Manfredi. "Not just certain European models, but the whole line," he reiterated. "I've proven my ability to sell DeManto automobiles. The *Professore* has made a lot of money, thanks to DonSport."

Manfredi translated for the Professor, and then translated the Old Man's reply: "The *Professore* says that he makes even more money from his existing American dealers."

"Which will doubtless continue," Morgan told Manfredi. "All I'm saying is that if necessary, my expanded network will be prepared to take up the slack should any of your existing dealers decide to bolt the fold."

The Italian went back and forth. Morgan took the opportunity to give Sonny an encouraging wink.

She was white-knuckled and twisting the hell out of her napkin, but she managed to respond with a faint smile.

"The *Professore* comments that your expanded network does not yet exist," Manfredi began. "The *Professore* asks what if he does these favors for you, his dealers desert him, and then your own network never gets off the ground?" There was triumph in Manfredi's voice as he said, "The *Professore* asks, what if you fail?"

This time Morgan addressed himself directly to the Old Man. "I don't fail. Not anymore. Not ever again."

The old fox knew more English than *he* let on. Morgan continued to speak directly to him, ignoring Manfredi, and even forgetting Sonny; forgetting that there was anyone else in the room beside himself and DeManto.

"Professore, a long time ago, in this very room, you told me that you were grateful for all I had done for your marque." He pointed to the sideboard. "For the trophies I've won for you. You told me then that you would live for the day when you could repay me by granting me a favor. That day has come. I'm here to request repayment of the favor."

The Professor rattled off something in Italian. Manfredi looked upset, but in the end he nodded respectfully, and stood up. "He wishes to speak to you two in private," Manfredi said, refusing to look Morgan in the eye, as he left the study, softly shutting the door behind him.

The Professor pushed himself away from the table, and then motioned to Morgan. "Donaldo, come closer," DeManto hoarsely whispered. Morgan obeyed, pulling up a dining room chair, so that they were face to face. "Donaldo . . ." the coal-black eyes glanced at Sonny. "Can she be trusted?"

"As her father could be," Morgan nodded.

DeManto cackled gleefully, showing stumps of ruined teeth. The sound was like night wind cutting through a graveyard. "Good . . . You're a lucky man, but then, you always been lucky, yes?" His tongue flicked out to lick the white spittle from his withered lips.

Morgan, staring into DeManto's knowing eyes felt a brush of panic. He knows. Somehow he found out about what really happened concerning Lee Thomas at Le Mans.

Thinking about it, Morgan realized that learning the truth about the incident wouldn't have been hard for someone like the Professor. DeManto could be relentless in pursuit of his quarry, and being who he was, he could have offered a lot to those involved. It would come as no surprise to Morgan that someone might have broken down and told DeManto the truth.

It would also be just like the Old Man to file the information away, saving it for a day when it could do him the most good—Morgan wondered if this was that day. How could he endure Sonny finally learning the truth in his presence, and from this man's lips?

"Donaldo, not a day has gone by in my life, I do not think about our last meeting. I think, did I do the right thing?" He nodded firmly. "For business, yes. But an old man learns there's more to life than business. You think you left me those cups," he pointed at the trophies, "so now I owe you a favor." He shook his head. "Those cups, they aren't a good reason." He held up his fingers in front of Morgan's face. "Those cups, they are as cold as my hands, and soon my hands will be just as dead, yes?" He laughed bitterly. "Donaldo, all my life I worship fast and powerful machines." The old man's gnarled finger hammered Morgan's knee for emphasis. "And my ambitions, they have all been realized." For just an instant, the coal-black eyes in the center of that wrinkled face lost their expressionless glitter; for an instant Morgan could see the frightened, lonely man trapped inside the legend. "Donaldo," the Professor whispered. "Machines cannot love back—"

DeManto plaintively gazed at Morgan, and must have seen the perplexed, helpless confusion that Morgan felt, because the old man abruptly shook himself, like a sleeper startled awake, and at once the eerie, reptilian mask was back in place.

"Donaldo, you be a good boy, and go outside, yes? I want to talk with this lovely, young *signorina* . . ."

Morgan hesitated, glancing at Sonny, feeling uneasy at the idea of these two having a conversation without him, but what could he do but acquiesce?

Morgan nodded. "I'll be in the garden." He got up, and left the study, not looking back. No one was around out in the hall. Morgan felt as if he and Sonny and the Professor were all alone in the big house.

He went downstairs and out the front door, then walked around to the garden, where he turned to look back at the ivy covered mansion, and high up, the glimmering, lit windows of the Professor's study. Sonny had been wrong, he decided. The massive fortress wasn't spooky, but it *was* haunting. You were awed by its magnificence, but something about the place also stirred a kind of pity for the man who had interred himself behind all that stone.

Would Morgan ever forget the look in DeManto's eyes when he'd said that machines can't love you back? And what was he supposed to make of it, Morgan wondered? Was it a dying old man's frightened plea for affection, or was it a warning?

How did the Professor know that Morgan had nothing in his own life to keep him going but his business—and his past? Sometimes Morgan thought he lived exclusively for his past . . .

Morgan glanced at his watch. Where was Sonny? Assuming the worst, that the canny Old Man *did* know the truth about what had really happened concerning Lee Thomas at Le Mans, would he tell Sonny? Was she going to come rampaging downstairs and into the garden to spit in Morgan's face?

And what about the damned deal? It would be just like the sardonic old bastard to agree to the deal and also see to it that it could never come to fruition by destroying Morgan's reputation, all in the space of a single afterdinner chat.

He found himself transfixed by those lit, study windows, and what might be unfolding behind them. What *were* DeManto and Sonny talking about? It galled Morgan to realize that once again his fate, and really his entire life, was resting in the gnarled hands of an old invalid.

Morgan was still in the garden, wandering among the ruined statues, playing tag with his memories, when Sonny found him.

"What did he want to talk to you about?" Morgan asked tensely.

"He just wanted to know if I was taking care of you," she lightly replied. "Keeping you off the sauce, stuff like that," Sonny finished.

"That's goddamned embarrassing," Morgan complained.

"Why look at it that way?" Sonny said. "He means well. He said that he feels like a father to you."

"That old bastard?" Morgan laughed curtly. "Remember what Manfredi said: DeManto's never felt like a father to anything that didn't have twelve cylinders."

"Well, you know him, I don't," Sonny shrugged. "But I think you're being unduly harsh."

"Bet your ass, I know him," Morgan nodded. "The Old Man has never done a goddamned thing that wasn't out of self-interest."

"Okay, then figure that DeManto wanted to know if

163

you had your act together for his own protection," Sonny agreed. "I think that's fair, Morgan. You're asking a lot of him: to commit himself to supplying DonSport America with vehicles, maybe antagonizing his existing dealer network; and to put his personal prestige on the line in coaxing the other Italian manufacturers to follow his lead." She shrugged. "Considering all that, I think he's got a right to know what the chances are of you folding, leaving him out on a limb."

Morgan turned to confront her. "You do, huh?" he demanded sternly.

Sonny flinched, but stood her ground. "Yes, I do."

"Well," he said, "what did you tell the Professor? Am I 'together'?"

"Morgan, how could you wonder?" she scolded him. "We're business partners. If I had to, I would have lied on your behalf."

"But you didn't have to lie?"

"Only partially. I mean, I know you don't drink. But something is wrong; I know it, I just don't know what it is."

"It doesn't concern you," Morgan said.

"Oh, sure it does," Sonny sighed. "In ways that I can guess, and in ways I can't." She hesitated. "The Professor told me about you when you were younger."

Morgan froze. Here it comes, he thought. DeManto's coup de grace.

"We started out talking about my father, but before long we'd segued over to you," Sonny said. "The Professor really likes you, Morgan. He really does—"

"I'm touched," Morgan said dryly.

"—But according to him, not as much as my father loved you."

"I really don't need to hear this." Why couldn't she get it over with, he wondered? Was she stretching it out in order to prolong his suffering?

"Yeah, you do," Sonny said flatly. "You know what the Professor told me? That my father felt like a father towards *you,* which is something I had kind of already remembered from my childhood. The Professor also said that fathers make sacrifices for their kids." She paused. "Do you have any idea what he meant by that, Morgan?"

Morgan was sweating. Could it be the Professor hadn't told her? But if DeManto knew the truth, why had he kept it a secret from Sonny? Unless, of course, Morgan's imagination was running amok, and the Professor's remarks about Morgan's luck, and fathers sacrificing for their children, were only the sort of vague cliches old men came up with to make conversation. Morgan just didn't know, and not knowing was making him feel crazy. It was all whirling and twirling around in his aching brain, along with his previous, gnawing obsession to know who had leaked his original plans to "Viewpoint."

"Morgan, you look like you're in such pain," Sonny sadly mourned, clutching at his hand. "Please let me help you."

"Sonny, there's nothing you can do." That much, at least, was true. The past was on his shoulders. Nobody could help him.

"It's getting late," Morgan said. "And who knows how late the Old Man stays up. We'd better go back inside. I'd like an answer from him before we leave."

"Wait. Sit down for a minute," she told him, gesturing toward a marble bench. "There's something I want to say," Morgan sat down and waited. "This isn't easy for me," she began, "so bear with me, and please don't interrupt. I know you've felt awful since I . . . well, tried to seduce you, a couple of nights ago," she swallowed, looking away. "Since then I've felt childish and stupid, and I've tried to compensate for my feelings by going to the opposite extreme. I know that my behavior has hurt you."

"It's okay, Sonny, you don't have to say anymore."

"But I want to," she insisted. "And here in this place

where my father spent so much time, I think that maybe I can find the strength, so please let me try."

"Okay," Morgan nodded. He looked around, noticed a fountain several paces away, and flashed on the fact that Lee Thomas had led him to this very bench on that long ago night when he'd offered Morgan the position of back-up driver.

For an instant, Morgan thought he could hear the Irishman's laughter, and the screech of a Formula One's fat black tires leaving rubber on the asphalt just before bouncing off of a guardrail and cartwheeling into flame . . . but it had to be just the rising night breeze rustling the branches, whistling around the eroded statuary.

"What happened that night in the hotel won't ever happen again, Morgan. That I promise you," Sonny declared. "I won't ever again allow my emotions to come between us. I guess we're not meant to be in love . . ."

She trailed off. Morgan thought that perhaps she was waiting for him to protest, to rescue her from her heartbroken misery. That was too bad; he was not a hero and a rescuer, and he never had been. Oh, he'd tried it once, with Ilsa, and he'd learned.

"Okay, so we're not meant to be lovers," Sonny plunged bravely on. "We do still have a lot in common . . ."

"Please, stop," Morgan said.

"Because we're so much alike, because we both love the same things, and because, in spirit, we're both my father's children, I just want you to know that we can be friends and partners, and that we can be easy in our relationship. Okay?"

Morgan looked at her. "Your father would have been very proud of you," he said. "I'm very proud of you."

Sonny chuckled. She kissed him on the cheek. "Well, I guess that'll have to do."

Morgan got up. "Come on, I want to get DeManto's decision."

"I already have it," Sonny gleefully announced. "He told me before I came out to see you. He's going to help us, Morgan." Her eyes were alight with triumph. "He'll participate in the race, and he'll use his clout to see to it that the other manufacturers participate as well."

_____ **13**

THAT NIGHT, MORGAN and Sonny drove back to their hotel. They were too excited to sleep, and sat up making future business plans. Sonny crashed around dawn. She dragged off to her room after making Morgan promise to let her sleep late that morning. Morgan dozed off as well, but woke early. By quarter to nine he was showered, shaved, and packed. He called down to room service for some breakfast, and at the stroke of nine called Fabiano Manfredi in order to firm up the details concerning the Professor's cooperation.

"_Buon giorno,_ Donaldo," Manfredi's voice came booming over the line after his secretary had put Morgan through. "The _Professore_ has informed me of his decision. It would be hypocritical of me to say that I'd initially approved, but now that we are committed, I congratulate you and wish you good fortune in this endeavor, my friend. I sincerely hope that this one time my business instincts will be proved wrong."

"Thank you, Fabi. There's no hard feelings on my part." Morgan thought Manfredi sincerely meant to mend fences. There was no question that Manfredi was devoted to the Professor, and would do his utmost to carry out the Old Man's wishes. "All I'm looking to do is make heaps of money for DonSport and DeManto."

"The _Professore_ wishes a few days in which to diplomatically broach the matter of your proposed publicity race to his business associates in order to bring them around to your point of view."

"I know that he can be a most charming and persuasive fellow," Morgan paused theatrically, "When it suits his purpose."

Manfredi chuckled. "Well, there are no guarantees in life, Donaldo, but I think it is safe for you to assume that with someone as prestigious as the *Professore* in your corner, the others' participation is assured."

"What should I be doing?"

"The *Professore's* instructions to you are simple: do nothing for the time being. You should not contact the other Italian manufacturers—not even to review their model lines. According to the *Professore*, these others are like children whom one must flatter and cajole— and if necessary dare—into doing as one wishes."

"Please inform the Professor that I will do exactly as he says. Please add that I am excited, and very grateful."

There was a pause on the other end of the line. "Perhaps it is the *Professore* who should be grateful to you, Donaldo," Manfredi quietly said. "I know that I am. I love him very much, and I know that he has fondness in his heart for me . . ."

"You are like a son to him, Fabi," Morgan said, trying his best to be diplomatic, although he had not altered his opinion from the night before that DeManto was incapable of loving anything that did not come equipped with bucket seats.

"I try to be," Manfredi said, sounding pleased, "But I think that he loves you even more."

Morgan was truly mystified. "Fabi, I haven't seen the Old Man in over a decade."

"I only know what I see, Donaldo, and what I feel in my heart. Perhaps the circumstances of your parting have weighed heavily on the *Professore* . . . If not for the entire time, certainly since his illness worsened, and he was forced to face his own mortality. Perhaps he began to wish that he could somehow make it up to you before he passed away." There was a pause during which Morgan could picture Manfredi's classic, philosophical shrug. "I only know that this morning the *Professore* was like a new man," Manfredi continued excitedly. "Today he went outside to the garden for a breath of fresh air, and he even left his wheelchair briefly."

"That is wonderful to hear," Morgan said, pleased. "I wish him a long life to come."

"Ah, who doesn't, Donaldo?" Manfredi sighed. "But we know that he can never fully regain his health. And yet, at the very least, his time remaining can be made more pleasurable. I did not know how to accomplish this, Donaldo, but you have managed to show me."

Morgan felt touched. "Fabi, all I've done is to give him the opportunity to pay back a little of what he thinks he owes me. Maybe the Professor's like me. I don't believe that a man can atone for his sins by making peace with God, but only by squaring his accounts with the people he's touched in life."

Manfredi was quiet for a beat. "Where did you come by your wisdom, my friend?"

"It was bought and paid for, Fabi," Morgan said wearily. "Bought and paid for."

"Well, for what you've accomplished, even if it was inadvertent, I thank you, Donaldo, on the *Professore*'s behalf, and on my own. In the years to come I look forward to continuing our business relationship, and our friendship."

"I would like that, too," Morgan said. "I'll call you in a few days, to see how the Old Man's made out." He broke the connection.

Morgan ate breakfast outside on the terrace, and then telephoned a cable to Niles Kingman in Paris, filling him in on the good news, and promising to keep him posted on further developments. By then it was

10:00. Morgan phoned Sonny's room. She answered on the fifth ring, her voice drugged with sleep. He told her to order up some breakfast and be ready to check out in an hour and a half.

"What's the rush?" she complained in muffled tones, as if her face was pressed against the pillows.

"It's a beautiful day, and I want to get on the road," Morgan enthused. He filled her in on his conversation with Fabiano Manfredi. "So that means we have a few days in which to do nothing but play," he said.

"Where we going?" Sonny demanded. The good news from Manfredi, and Morgan's good mood, had seemed to perk her up.

"Eden," Morgan joked. "Or as close as we can come to Eden in this day and age."

"Does that mean I can regain my lost innocence?" Sonny joked.

"Well, I suppose it's never too late," Morgan said.

"That's what I've been trying to tell *you,*" Sonny said, and hung up.

"It's so funny to me that you would have a villa in Portofino," Sonny told Morgan once they and their luggage were settled in the Scorpio, and they were on the road. "It's so unlike you. I mean, everything about you is so spartan—"

"That's not true," Morgan protested.

"Of course it is," Sonny waved him quiet. "Name one thing you indulge in that has nothing to do with business."

"Clothes—"

"A business expense. You'd wear jeans and running shoes all the time if you could. Name something else."

"Food," Morgan said slowly, "and . . ."

"And what?" Sonny challenged, laughing.

"Well, I suppose I see your point," Morgan admitted mildly. He shrugged. "Anyway, the villa is certainly just for fun. I bought the place just after I was married.

171

It became sort of our getaway. After my wife died, I just hung onto it. It's very laid-back," he glanced at Sonny. "There are no servants, or anything like that."

"No servants!" Sonny pretended to be horrified. "I don't know about you, Morgan. No wonder Robin Leach hasn't called you . . ."

"I don't know what you're expecting," Morgan laughed, "but I hope you're not disappointed. The place was built in the sixteenth century, and it needed work *then*. There's just a caretaker from the village to check up on the place, and try to maintain it, you know, pick up the biggest pieces as they fall off. I phoned him from the hotel to let him know we're coming, so the place should be aired out, and stocked with provisions. We've been eating in restaurants so much, I thought I'd cook tonight. Tomorrow we'll reserve a table at Puny's."

"I am so psyched for this," Sonny said happily. "But you still haven't told me how you ended up with a villa in the first place—Wait! Don't tell me!" She thought hard. "You *won* it! That's it!" she exalted. "You won it from . . . an Italian count—and I bet he was a handsome devil—you won it by beating him in a high speed, cliff-hanging, one-on-one sports car race . . . On this very road."

"Actually, I bought it from this Jewish guy in New York," Morgan said. "I met him through my business manager. He was in the garment business—men's clothing—so I endorsed one of his lines. This was back in the early seventies, you realize . . . Well, the poor guy paid a fortune for the villa, figuring to tear it down and start all over. He didn't know that you can't do so much as cut down a tree in Portofino, let alone put up a Malibu beach house, or whatever he had in mind. But I guess the straw that broke the camel's back was the fact that Portofino has a pretty laid-back nightlife. No discos, or anything; not back then, and not now. You can't even take a car into the village. Well, to make a long story short, he almost paid me to take it off of his hands." Morgan shrugged. "When I was married I used it a lot; now I'm here once or twice a year." He paused. "The place holds a lot of memories—"

"You don't say?" Sonny drawled, and Morgan glared at her, affronted by her sarcastic tone.

"Look, Morgan, I know you're into brooding and all. You're kind of like a Byron type, you know?"

"Uh-huh." He fought to keep a straight face. If he laughed, he might not get to hear what else she was going to say.

"Now, that introspective thing is cool. . . . I guess a lot of women find that sort of thing sexy, but it's not really my style. If we're going to be working together, you might as well know that I'm a today kind of person. I'm not into the past. I care about the future."

"Uh-huh, okay," Morgan said dryly. "I'll keep all that in mind. Anyway, the villa is where I go to unwind."

Sonny laughed. "That I can't *wait* to see."

Morgan made good time along the A1 autostrada, leaving it a few kilometers past Parma, where he switched to the A15 for a straight run to the Ligurian sea. At the trading port of La Spézia they picked up the Via Aurelia, the central artery through the Riviera Di Levante.

At La Spézia the road curved inland, past ancient stone walls laced with flowering vines, through sun-dappled stands of pine and cypress and along hills blanketed with olive groves. They stopped at a small, sunbaked village to buy picnic provisions from the stall vendors lining the tiny, dusty square, where several weathered old gentlemen in worn work clothes were holding court over a bottle of wine at a modest, outdoor taverna. Morgan and Sonny bought bread, cheese, and peaches, and for Sonny, a half liter of Conqueterra, the straw-colored, sweet white wine named for the nearby Five Lands area, where the men were lowered on ropes to harvest the grapes from the cliffside vines. Morgan bought bottled orangeade for himself, and they set out again, anxious to catch their first glimpse of the sea.

At the resort town of Sestri Levante, the road finally met the coast. They ate their picnic lunch at a turnoff a little further along, spreading out their food on a rocky ledge at the foot of a desolate, crumbling, medieval watchtower above the placid blue sea.

From Sestri Levante it was relatively slow going along the winding, narrow road. Since the weather was mild and sunny, they slid back the Scorpio's sunroof, and lowered the windows to enjoy the sound of the waves crashing against the rocky shoreline, and the mingled fragrances of the sea and the inland groves of ripening oranges and lemons. Morgan maneuvered the Scorpio through the tangle of cars and lollipop-colored Vespas swarming around the overblown tourist meccas of Chiávari and Rapallo, with their public beaches and daytripper sightseeing voyages, and at long last, onto the Portofino Peninsula, where the road once again left the ocean. It was now late in the afternoon. Morgan drove hard and fast, anxious to be there in time for the sunset. He glanced at Sonny now and then. She seemed content to lie back against the Scorpio's glove leather seat, basking in the warmth, and enjoying the scenic stands of pine and palm flying by.

At last Morgan saw the signposts for Portofino. A few hundred yards before coming to the village proper, he turned onto a dirt road that wended its way up through a thickly wooded hillside, and then he turned off onto a still narrower road—really just a rutted mule track that corkscrewed its way up the cliffs. And then they were there. He eased the car through a high, wrought iron gate into a small, bricked courtyard, enclosed on the left by a wall of vegetation. The courtyard's second and third walls were formed by the mossy, gray stone sides of the L-shaped villa. There was a low wing, with a steeply pitched, terra-cotta tiled roof. There were lots of narrow, arched, shuttered windows, and rough-hewn wooden doors with elaborate, rusted iron hinges. The main part of the house was three stories tall, with the same sort of roof. Capping it was a narrow, rounded tower, the width of one room, like a castle's battlement.

Morgan shut off the engine. At once they were engulfed in a peaceful silence broken only by birdsong, the buzz of insects, and, from the villa's far side, the faint crash of water against rock.

Morgan turned to Sonny and grinned. "Welcome to Portofino."

As they were getting out of the car, Pietro, the caretaker, appeared from around a corner to greet them. He was short and stocky in baggy chinos, and an off-white cotton crewneck sweater. He had the chunky shoulders and thick arms that came from a lifetime spent hauling nets from out of the sea.

Morgan introduced Pietro to Sonny; the Italian nodded shyly, unable or unwilling to look her in the eye as he shook hands with her. Morgan saw that Sonny looked slightly thrown by the Italian's uncertain welcome. Morgan winked at her and told her not to take offense; Pietro was shy around all women.

He asked his caretaker if preparations had been made for them. As was always the case, between Morgan's broken Italian and Pietro's fractured English, they were able to meet somewhere in the linguistic middle ground and communicate. Pietro told Morgan that he'd stocked the larder according to orders, that there were clean towels and linens in the closets, and that everything else was in more or less working order.

"Well, time to show you around," Morgan told Sonny as Pietro unloaded their car. "This low wing is closed off. I just used the main part of the house. It's two floors, and then there's the tower, which gives me another two rooms, one stacked on top of the other. He led her inside, nudging open the wood framed screen door with his foot. It was really just one big room, about fifty feet long and thirty feet wide, with a kitchen area at one end, a steep narrow staircase leading upstairs off to the right, and a set of glass doors at the far side. The floor was worn gray stone, the ceiling was low and crisscrossed with massive, honey colored rafters, the walls were rough stucco, but brightly whitewashed.

"Morgan, this is just like your apartment in San Francisco!" Sonny laughed.

"Gee, you know, I never thought of that. I guess you're right." Out of the corner of his eye Morgan saw a black shape dart past and scamper up the staircase. "That's Felix," he told Sonny.

"As in 'cat'?"

Morgan nodded. "He keeps the mouse population down to a dull roar." He looked at her, concerned. "You're not going to freak out over a few cute little mice, right?"

"Italian mice? How chic . . ." she bravely declared.

Morgan laughed. He pointed at a door leading off of the kitchen. "That's the bathroom. Only one where you can actually bathe, I'm afraid. The kitchen stove runs on propane, as does the hot water heater." He looked sheepish. "You'll find it's best to make showers short and sweet. The hot water heater is truly Italian in temperment. This whole place will probably get blown to smithereens one of these days."

"If it does while I'm here, I'll die with a smile on my face," Sonny told him. "So far I think everything is great."

Morgan nodded, feeling unaccountably pleased. "Well, I like it, and I'm glad you do, too," he added shyly, suddenly feeling just like poor tongue-tied Pietro. He watched Sonny take in the rest of the room: the huge fireplace; the grouping of white enameled metal furniture—patio furniture, really—with cushions upholstered in bright red canvas; the eclectic collection of lamps and side tables, the floor-to-ceiling bookcase loaded with volumes.

"There's not much to do here . . ." Morgan said as he watched Sonny scan the titles. He watched, grinning with anticipation, as Sonny moved to the glass doors.

"Oh, my god, Morgan!"

Morgan followed her as she threw open the doors and stepped out onto the wide, brick terrace. Its worn, stone balustrades were covered over with vines, while bougainvilleas and roses grew in long, low, stone planters. Morgan led her to the edge, where a break in the balustrade offered access to a zigzagging stone stairway. It led down some 100 feet to the water lapping gently against a stone pier, to which was tied a small sailboat. Off to their right lay the opalescent Bay of Tiguillo, dotted with more sailboats, its far horizons lost in haze. Directly across from the villa, separated from it by the narrow inlet that served as the marina, was pastel-shaded Portofino, gently curved like a sliver of crescent moon around the deep blue water.

"Come on, I'll show you the upstairs." He managed to tear her away from the view and back into the house, then up the steep staircase. "Mind your head as you go up and down," he warned her. "They didn't grow people very tall in the sixteenth century."

The upstairs was divided up, two rooms to a floor, separated by the narrow landing. The rooms were done pretty much in the simple, utilitarian style of the downstairs: whitewashed walls, straw mats on the worn wooden floors, a junk shop mix of lamps, canvas slung chairs, and futon couches. The top floor held a pair of bedrooms, with mirrored bureaus and double beds. All the rooms had views of the water.

Stuck between the bedrooms, formed from space borrowed from both of them, was a small lavette.

"It took months to get the building permits and cost a small fortune to run the pipes, but it sure beats running up and down these steps in the middle of the night. I'm into roughing it," Morgan explained, "but I'm not crazy."

There was a fireplace in each room. Morgan told her that woodfires were the only means of heating the villa, but not to worry because it never got that cold on the Ligurian coast due to the southern exposure and the hills that sheltered it from the north winds. Anyway, he had lots of sweaters to loan.

He took her up to the tower, via a relatively new, metal, circular stairway. "I got tired of the ladder," Morgan explained. At the base of the narrow tower he showed her the doors that led out to the third floor roof terrace, which also offered a view of the water and the village.

"Where are your neighbors?" Sonny asked, following Morgan back downstairs. "You can't own all this much land, can you?"

"Oh, there are little places like mine tucked in all over the place, but it's all pretty private. It's the guys with the big, luxurious villas who have to worry about sticking out like a bald spot."

They changed into shorts and light cotton sweaters, the only clothes they'd need in Portofino, Morgan told her; and from the third floor terrace they watched the setting sun, the size and color of a blood orange suspended in a violet sky, send bolts of scarlet across the water. At some point Sonny silently moved close to Morgan, and he put his arm around her.

It was just a familial gesture, he told himself. A hug between friends was all it was. There was no need to sweat it, to let the bad memories intrude on this blissful, innocent moment. Anyway, it was damned *good* to hold her close, and pretend, for just a little while, that there was no nasty secret to keep them apart. When, finally, the red sun dipped below the shimmering horizon, it was Sonny who, with a seemingly knowing, seemingly satisfied smile, pulled away from him.

They went inside where Morgan gave her a glass of wine, and she kept him company in the kitchen. She tended to the fireplace while he fixed them a dinner of scampi made with succulent, coral pink prawns, and a green salad, accompanied by a huge loaf of crusty bread. They finished off the remains of the bread with gorgonzola, and some peaches, followed by espresso. After dinner, Morgan suggested they go outside to sit by the water. Sonny took her wine, and Morgan lit a candle to show them their way across the terrace and down the old stone steps to the water's edge. It was a balmy night, slightly humid, but the sky was clear, moonless, and full of stars. Across the inlet, the waterside restaurants and taverns of Portofino glittered with small lights, like fireflies.

They sat on old blankets, dangled their bare feet in the cool water gently lapping at the stone pilings, and talked. For a while they talked of the future, of hard, business matters, but before long Sonny had Morgan talking about Lee Thomas. It seemed to him that she could never hear enough about her father. Morgan tried to oblige her. At first he felt uneasy. This was dangerous territory. Then Morgan realized that what Sonny wanted to hear about was her father's *life*, not his death. Fueled by her delighted laughter he spun countless tales of his wild times with Lee Thomas.

An hour passed, then two, then three. The candle had long since sputtered, and as they talked and laughed, the lights of Portofino began to blink out one by one, until it seemed to Morgan that he and Sonny were all alone by the onyx water, beneath a thousand crystal stars.

They'd run out of talk. Morgan was lying on his back, gazing at the sky, listening to the creaking of the little sailboat as it rose and fell on the water. Sonny was curled up beside him, her head on his chest. He was gently stroking her hair when she pushed herself up and looked into his eyes, and then he was twisting around in their warm nest of soft blankets in order to kiss her.

Her mouth tasted of wine, and he couldn't help thinking that the taste was an omen that this woman was *twice* forbidden to him.

But she felt so good, and he couldn't stop kissing her, and her hands were sliding beneath his shorts—

He pulled away from her. She tried to pull him back, but he brushed her arm away, a trifle roughly, perhaps. He sat with his back to her, at the very edge of the stone embankment, with his feet dangling in the water. *To cool off,* he thought. He could hear her breathing.

"Morgan?" Her voice was light, but he heard traces of doubt, and anger.

"There's something you have to know, before we . . ."

"Enough talk, Morgan, it's time to put up and shut up," she tried to joke.

"It's about your father and me. You have to know what happened."

"All right, talk to me."

And so I will, Morgan realized. *Holy shit. I really will—*

"I was in a very bad way when your father rehired me," Morgan began, a part of him thinking that this couldn't really be him speaking—*confessing*. "This was right after my wife's death, you see. I guess you know she died of a drug overdose . . . I tried to help her to beat her habit, but I was very naive. I thought that if I loved her enough, everything would be all right," he laughed ruefully. "Like I said, I was very naive." As he spoke, he kept his back to Sonny, looking out over the water toward the dark village. He took his time; examining each word as it came out of his mouth as if it were an ancient artifact, packed away years ago, now unwrapped from its moldering cloth and held up to the light. If this was a confession, he intended to do it right and wash himself clean in exchange for paying the painful price. "I guess at that point I already had a drinking problem. For a while I laid off the booze, but it was too late to save my ride with DeManto. With no job, and Ilsa gone, well, I just didn't have any focus; everything seemed meaningless." Morgan shrugged. "So I started in again drinking. A lot. There was no way anybody was going to let me drive for them, but I did manage to wrangle a job as a commentator on one of the networks covering the Grand Prix circuit. They put me in this blazer with their insignia on the breast pocket and trotted me out now and then for what they called 'color commentary'."

"I remember," Sonny said. "I remember how very handsome you looked on TV," she added softly.

"It was a stupid job, but it paid a little, and it gave me a reason to stay on the racing circuit. Before long though, I'd screwed myself out of it. I showed up drunk for a broadcast, and they took away my pretty blazer with the insignia. I still traveled from one Grand Prix site to the other. It was all I knew. I wasn't even thirty years old, but I was a has-been. I was a joke. Like the ex-great-gunfighter turned town drunk in all those western flicks."

"That's when my father found you?"

"Yeah. You know, a little bit after I'd gotten my own ride with DeManto, and I was at the top, your father and I had a falling out. I guess I was full of myself, and maybe your father was a little overbearing, but whatever the cause, we ended our friendship and stopped speaking. But when I was down on my luck, there was Lee to offer me a helping hand."

"That was my dad," she said proudly.

"Lee literally pulled me out of the gutter," he told her. "He forced me to get my act together. He told me that if I could stay sober, he'd give me a ride as one of his back-up drivers." Morgan swiveled around to face Sonny. She was seated cross-legged on the blankets, leaning slightly toward him, her mouth a thin, straight line as she listened intently. It was too dark to see her eyes. Morgan was very grateful for that.

"So you sobered up," Sonny said. "You took the ride."

"God help me, Sonny, I took it."

She shook her head. "I'm sorry to be so dense, but I still don't understand what's bothering you so . . ."

Morgan took a deep breath and let it out slowly. "You will . . ." He ran his hand through his hair, then went on. "Anyway, you can imagine how I felt when your father, without an ounce of recrimination, offered me that ride as a back-up driver. I'd had a lot on my shoulders, but I let it all fall away. I kind of regressed, I guess; I tried to recapture my youth as a member of Lee's circus, with no responsibilities but to hone my skills behind the wheel of that big brute of a racing green BXI Formula One. I almost succeeded."

"What do you mean?" Sonny asked quietly.

"I wasn't drinking," Morgan said. "Honestly, I wasn't touching a drop. No wine, no beer; nothing. And I was driving every day, but it was gone, Sonny. Whatever natural ability I'd had behind the wheel was gone. Call it talent, or genius . . ." Morgan looked away. "Whatever it was, I'd lost it. I was petrified that your father would find out and fire me. Here I was back safe and sound in the extended family of the circus, beneath your father's paternal wing. The last thing I wanted was to be cast out of that nest a second time. So I pretended to practice, and I sweated every race, afraid that he'd tell me to drive a lap or two, and see that I was incapable of doing anything but stroking it."

"I remember that BXI was constantly on my dad's ass about you," Sonny said. "They didn't think you had it any longer."

Morgan nodded. "And they were right. Anyway, Lee never did ask me to drive. Partly it was dumb luck, I guess."

"And you were the newest back-up," Sonny added. "There would have been plenty of others in the circus with seniority," she smiled fondly, "on those few occasions when my hot-foot of a dad felt indisposed."

"Your father drove every race," Morgan agreed. "He was still one of the best, but he was getting older, and maybe he'd begun to wonder how many seasons he had left. All the other teams were fielding much younger drivers with the sharper reflexes and increased stamina that come from youth." Morgan shrugged. "Well, it went on like that, with your father flogging himself to keep up with drivers half his age. Lee was doing okay, but not up to his previous levels of performance. BXI began to give him some flack."

"I didn't know that," Sonny said.

"You wouldn't have," Morgan replied. "Your mom probably didn't, either. It wasn't like your father to share his problems. I only knew about it because I was around when one of the BXI execs put your father through the wringer. Anyway, it was the beginning of the manufacturer's round of races. Your dad announced the schedule. He was very fair. Every back-up driver was to get to drive in a race. Including me. He'd assigned me the best of them: Le Mans. The other drivers were pissed off, but Lee was adamant. I was to be his relief driver at Le Mans. He said BXI wanted it that way: the media angle of the old team of Thomas/ Morgan, back and ready to kick ass at their favorite stomping grounds, blah-blah-blah." Morgan shook his head. "That was a load of crap, and everyone knew it. BXI thought I was yesterday's newspaper and would have been very happy if I dropped into a deep hole, never to be heard from again."

"My dad made you his relief for Le Mans because he loved you," Sonny stated flatly.

That was true, Morgan realized. Lee Thomas had loved him like a son. Morgan flashed on DeManto's comment, relayed to him by Sonny that night in the Old Man's garden: "*. . . fathers will sacrifice for their children . . .*" He was finally beginning to understand what the Professor had been trying to say to him that night. Maybe guilt and redemption wasn't as clear-cut as black and red profit and loss figures entered into the columns of some ledger. Lee Thomas had loved him, and he loved Lee: maybe that love counted for something against the burden of guilt and pain he'd been shouldering for so long?

The epiphany solaced Morgan, and gave him the strength to continue running this emotional gauntlet on Sonny's—and his own—behalf.

"That much about my father I'll always remember," Sonny went on. "He loved you, and maybe he figured that the two of you making a good showing at Le Mans would show the world that you were back. That you were once again ready for a ride of your own." She thought about it. "Maybe he was also doing it for himself, to a degree. Maybe he was hoping that with you behind him he could catch himself a piece of Indian Summer in the autumn of his career."

"I should have told Lee about my lack of confidence," Morgan said. "I should have leveled with him, but I was afraid to, Sonny. I was afraid that he'd fire me and I'd be back on my own, with no prospects and nothing to do but drink . . . I'd been on the wagon for about six months. By then, all the rah-rah enthusiasm about starting a new life had worn off. I was looking at spending the rest of my life straight, and it was awesome." Morgan stared at her silhouette in the darkness. "Sonny, you've got to understand: all I had was Lee Thomas and his circus. There was no way I could admit to him that I was incapable of driving."

"But . . . Morgan, I don't understand. You *did* drive . . ."

He hesitated. Now or never, he thought. He could still lie; still make up some story to keep her from hating him for the rest of her life.

"I didn't drive, Sonny." Morgan felt his eyes grow wet, heard his voice breaking. "I didn't drive . . ." He had to stop; he was having trouble breathing.

"For God's sake, Morgan," Sonny demanded, her voice low and urgent. "What happened?"

She was leaning towards him, her body taut; Morgan thought that she looked like some fierce predator about to pounce. *Lie-lie-lie,* his instincts howled, but for better or worse the festering lies were about to die a long deserved death.

"Sonny, the day of the race, while your father was driving that first stint, I freaked. I left the pit, went to a nearby tavern, and began to drink. Some of the crew found me. I was totally wrecked, so they left me there, with my head on the table, and my arms wrapped around a bottle. I was still there when the news swept the tavern that Lee Thomas had crashed and burned."

"What are you saying?" Sonny demanded, and then started to cry. "Morgan?"

"BXI had instituted cost-cutting measures. They hadn't let your father bring any other drivers to Le Mans. If he had to withdraw from the race because of me, his own reputation would have been destroyed, and maybe BXI would have fired him."

"He drove your stint, didn't he?" Sonny's voice was harsh. "Answer me, you bastard! My father, dead tired after driving his own stint, went back out there pretending he was *you*. And then he had to drive a *third* straight stint, his own."

"Yes," Morgan whispered. "Much later, Sonny, after the accident, and after I'd sobered up, the chief mechanic told me that the accident would never have happened if Lee hadn't been so totally fatigued. *'Driver's error,'* the mechanic sneered at me, with such hatred and contempt in his eyes. *'Driver's error,'* he said, *'and we all know what Lee's error was, don't we?'* "

Morgan saw Sonny's clenched fists. He was doubly grateful for the darkness, so that he did not have to see that same hatred and contempt that had been in the mechanic's eyes in her own.

"How did the truth stay a secret so long?" she demanded. "How did you manage to walk away clean from this?"

"Only the pit crew and I knew that your father had pretended to be me. I wasn't about to tell—"

"But dammit, why did the crew protect *you?*"

"They didn't. At least, that wasn't their primary intention. The crew were loyal to your father. If they spilled the secret of how he'd broken the rules, his entire career would have been overshadowed. He was dead; they wanted to let him go out a hero. They kept the secret for *Lee,* not for me."

"I understand . . . *now,*" Sonny coldly replied.

"I never touched another drop of alcohol after that awful day. A little while after, I got the idea for DonSport. I made a few appointments with the European car manufacturers, and then, in California, I used my old jet set contacts to spread the word to my potential clientele. DonSport, Ltd. was born." Morgan hesitated. "Your family shared in the first dollar I made, Sonny."

She nodded. "You made it *seem* like you were honoring a business partnership with my father, but that partnership never existed, did it?" Sonny asked curtly. "All you were trying to do with your money was . . . *atone!*" she accused.

"Yes." Morgan felt numb now.

"And what about *my* job, Morgan?" she asked, her voice dripping with sarcasm. "The job I have now, and my future place in DonSport America? Is all of that more *atonement* on your part?"

"Sonny, you know better than that—"

"I don't know anything at all. I sure as hell don't know *you,* do I? I thought I did, but I was wrong! You've tried to make things up with money, but all the money in the world can't give me back my father, can it, Morgan?" her voice was cruel.

"No . . . Money can't bring him back. Nothing can, but there hasn't been a day I haven't regretted what I did, Sonny. Even now, if there was any way I could trade my life for his; anyway I could go back and wipe away that accident—"

"*No,*" Sonny snapped. "*Not* accident. *Murder.* What happened to Lee Thomas had nothing to do with chance. You *killed* him."

"Sonny, you don't mean that!" Morgan shouted as he watched her get to her feet and hurry up the stairs back to the villa. He stood up to follow her, but at the top of the stairs she turned, to point a rigid finger down at him.

"Don't come near me, Morgan," she whispered harshly. "I'm warning you, stay away. Just—*stay away from me!*"

He watched as she disappeared into the villa. He stayed where he was, wondering if she were up there crying, or was she rummaging through the kitchen drawers right now, selecting the meanest, sharpest butcher knife with which to come hurtling down the stairs, an avenging fury?

The phrase *not worth killing* went through Morgan's mind, but he decided that he was probably being overly modest—

And then he laughed, because after so many years, he was all cried out. And because nobody could hurt him more than he'd hurt himself.

And then, because the heart and soul and conscience are the most cantankerous things, he curled up into a fetal position on those soft blankets and went to sleep. And it was the deepest, darkest, most peaceful sleep that he'd had in years.

14

HE WOKE TO the raucous chatter of quarreling gulls. His watch said 8:00 A.M. The sun was bright, the sky was clear blue, and across the inlet the quays of Portofino were already alive with strollers. Morgan watched a carnation pink sailboat cast off. Its auxiliary outboard motor sent up blue smoke a second before the buzz came traveling over the water. The sailboat pulled away from the dock, made a tight turn, and cruised the inlet too fast, furrowing a deep wake that sent waves slapping up against Morgan's stone embankment, splashing him. He watched the sailboat put out to the open water of the bay. It cut its motor and hoisted a white sail that filled immediately with wind. It merged with the other taut sails that from this distance reminded Morgan of stately swans.

He sat up and stretched. He felt eyes upon him and turned towards the stairs. Sonny, in tan shorts and a red, DonSport T-shirt, her long dark hair still damp from the shower, sat watching him. She looked pale and haggard. There were deep shadows under her eyes. She looked like she hadn't slept.

"How long have you been out here?" Morgan asked timidly, not knowing what kind of response to expect.

"An hour. I checked your room, but you weren't there."

"I was here," Morgan needlessly explained. At least they were talking, and not screaming at each other.

"You stayed out here all night, huh?" she asked quietly. "Why?" When Morgan shrugged, she added, "Were you doing penance, or were you afraid to come into the house?"

"All of the above," he said. She kind of smiled, and his heart skipped a beat as hope surged. "You look like you had a rough night as well."

"I did," Sonny nodded. "I didn't sleep at all. When I ran into the house last night I hated you. I prowled around my bedroom like some kind of psycho, cursing you, imagining a million horrible ways to murder you. I actually started packing my bags to leave."

"That would have done it," Morgan observed.

"Done what?"

"Murdered me," he said. She looked away. "If you'd left, it would have killed me . . ." he persisted. She stayed quiet. Morgan waited a moment, and then said, "But you didn't leave."

"No," Sonny softly agreed. "I'm still here."

Morgan took a deep breath. "Does that mean we're friends, again?"

"Friends . . ." Sonny echoed, trying the word out. She shook her head sadly. "What we are isn't so clear-cut, but then, it never was."

"Sonny—"

"Hush, let me talk. Last night, during my rage—as I cursed and plotted against you, I suddenly remembered something about what I was feeling that moment when my father died. I watched his death on television, you know . . . I remember the announcer's voice got really squeaky; he was talking a mile a minute, like the announcer on that newsreel footage of the *Hindenburg* explosion. I remember how I thought I wasn't understanding; that my daddy couldn't be dead." She looked away from Morgan, out toward the bay. She looked aloof, and serene, and very beautiful. "When it finally sank in, all during the time I was crying my heart out, I remember how some part of me was whispering that at least *you* were all right."

Morgan wanted to weep, but he had no tears left. "I can't cry anymore, Sonny," he said softly.

She pinned Morgan with her intense gaze. "You cried a long time," she said. "You've been crying all these years, during which you stuck by my family and me, when you really didn't have to. You've cried enough." She granted him a tired smile. "I guess I might have said some things last night that I didn't mean," Sonny continued. "Or maybe I meant them last night, but I don't now. I know that you didn't murder my father. You didn't put a gun to his head and make him drive. That was his choice."

"I let him down—"

"But you didn't kill him," Sonny insisted. "You've got to stop believing that you did. I understand now why you don't compete in races. I understand why you felt compelled to cook up this silly ruse concerning my driving for you at this publicity race at Le Mans. I'll still do it for you. I'll still be friends and business partners with you; as for anything else between us, I guess we'll have to see. And if you were asking for my forgiveness last night, I suppose you have it, but in return, you've got to do something for me."

"I'd do anything for you, Sonny . . ."

"Then let all this *go*," she urged. "My father's been dead a long time. Let him rest in peace, and get on with your life. If you want to honor my father, do it by *living*. Lee Thomas would have had it no other way." She abruptly began to cry, and just as suddenly stopped, sniffling loudly, and giving her nose a savage rub. "I guess all I know is that my father *believed* in you. I don't intend to let either one of us prove him wrong." She waited a moment, and then cocked her head, staring at Morgan. "Well, what do you have to say?"

"Did you make any coffee?"

Deadpan, Sonny said, "Yes, I made coffee. And I don't know how to make decent coffee, which means that the coffee is better than you deserve."

Morgan stood up and stretched. "You can't always get justice in this world."

They took the sailboat across the inlet and spent the morning in Portofino. Morgan showed Sonny the prettiest of the ancient, narrow alleyways lined with candy colored facades. There was some initial awkwardness between them, but it gradually dissipated.

They tried their damndest to find something to buy at the boutiques, but they couldn't. They already had everything they wanted—shorts, sweaters, sneakers—and for the first time, a mutual serenity that allowed them to pal around like an old married couple. Now that Morgan had finally let go of his secret, had revealed the worst to Sonny, and she had forgiven him, he felt far more at ease with her. It wasn't logical, but relationships rarely were. This was the gentle calm that lingers after a fierce storm. The build-up and release of nervous tension between them was almost like the build-up and release of sleeping together for the first time.

Except that they hadn't slept together, at least, not yet. Well, maybe that would come, no pun intended, Morgan thought. Or maybe not. Sonny would have to decide. This last, *very last* time she would have to make the first move. Morgan knew that if the lovemaking was to be any good, Sonny would have to resolve whatever contradictory feelings still lingered in her.

They ate a quick lunch and then took the sailboat out onto the bay for a couple of hours, tying up again in time to make the stroll to the little church of San Giorgio to watch the sunset. Back in the village they had a drink at a quayside cafe, and then went to dinner at Puny's, where they feasted on lasagne al pesto, calamari, and mussels steamed in white wine. By the time they got back to the villa they were like two stumbling, sleepy-eyed children up way past their bedtimes.

In bed, Morgan wished that Sonny were beside him.

He could hear her bed's creaking and groaning coming from across the hall, and wondered if she were wishing the same thing. He had almost rationalized to himself why it made sense for him to go knock on her door when he remembered what she'd said to him this morning about being friends and partners, but as for anything else, she'd have to see.

So he'd wait. But every time her damned bed creaked he stiffened—in more ways than one—thinking that he was about to hear her footsteps in the hall, and then the knock on his bedroom door.

He fell asleep waiting.

The next morning they packed a picnic, and made the five hour roundtrip hike along the well marked path from Portofino to the jewellike fishing village of San Fruttuoso. They got back to the villa, sunburned and tired, but proud of themselves, late in the afternoon. Sonny wanted a shower and a nap, so Morgan took the boat across the inlet to shop for dinner. When he got back Sonny was asleep on a chaise longue in the shaded area of the third floor terrace. Morgan went back to the kitchen. He cleaned and filleted the fish, put it in the fridge, then put the trimmings and shrimp shells into a pot with water, some white wine, and celery, and set it to simmering to make a stock. He chopped up the vegetables he'd bought, and was sauteeing onions and garlic in olive oil when the telephone, dusty and forgotten, began to ring.

He turned down the flame beneath the frying pan, and answered the phone. There was a sound like bacon frying, and then the operator, telling him it was long distance from the USA, and to stand-by.

"Hello, Don? Don Morgan? It's Joe Weiner."

"Joe! How are you?" Morgan said, surprised. He checked the time: five in the afternoon here in Italy, which was about ten hours ahead of West Coast time. "You're up and around pretty early."

"Specifically to talk to you," Weiner laughed. "Hear me okay?"

"Sure." The connection was clear and strong, except for that background of sizzling static.

"I got your number last night from your secretary," Weiner said. "I just about had to use torture to wring it out of her."

"I'm sorry about that, Joe," Morgan chuckled. "But Beth is very protective of my privacy."

Sonny, yawning and stretching, came down the stairs. "Who's that?" she asked.

Morgan silently mouthed *Joe Weiner* and Sonny, her eyebrows arched in bemusement, said, "Well, what do you know about that? . . ." She nosed about the steaming pots for a moment. Morgan kept an eye on her. He knew that when it came to cooking, she couldn't boil water. Then she went to the refrigerator to pour herself a glass of juice.

"What can I do for you, Joe?"

"Well, it's more what *I* want to do," Weiner said. "I want to apologize to you. I was positive that the leak concerning your expansion plans hadn't originated at Weiner, Carlson and Boyd. I was positive, and I was wrong. It *was* one of my employees—an ex-employee let me hasten to add—who talked to 'Viewpoint.' An investigation here on an entirely unrelated matter brought the situation to light. You see, the guy had been in charge of a deal we were about to do with Kingman and Son—"

"Bingo," Morgan said.

"Pardon me, Don?"

"Joe, was this guy's connection Niles Kingman?"

"Yes, until Niles Kingman abruptly walked away from the negotiations. I'm sure you understand that I can't go into the specifics of the deal. We were running a review to try and figure out what had caused the Kingman group's abrupt cold shoulder. That was when our employee panicked and confessed that he had leaked the info about you to Kingman in a stupidly misguided attempt to impress the man and clinch the deal. A few days later 'Viewpoint' contacted this employee, and in the best tradition of checkbook journalism, got him to tell the specifics." Weiner hesitated. "I talked to my lawyers about the possibility of reporting this guy and 'Viewpoint' to the proper authorities, but the advice I got was to let it go. My firm doesn't need that kind of publicity. If you think about it, I believe you'll come to the conclusion that DonSport doesn't want that sort of media attention, either."

"No, you're right, Joe," Morgan said. "I'm just relieved to know that it wasn't anyone from my company."

"I figured you would be. That's why I used the thumbscrews on your secretary. I didn't want to wait until you got back home to tell you. Once again, please accept my sincerest apologies for this mess . . ." Weiner again hesitated. "My attorneys have also pointed out to me that you'd be in your rights to sue our pants off . . ."

Morgan smiled. Weiner sounded very worried. "That's not going to happen, buddy. Like you said, it'd get very messy, and neither one of us wants that kind of publicity."

"Jeez," Weiner sighed. "I really owe you . . ."

"When I get back, you can buy me the world's most expensive lunch, okay?"

"Thanks, Don," Weiner said, sounding ultra-relieved. "I owe you one hell of a favor—"

"I'll call you when I get back," Morgan told him, and hung up the phone.

"What was that all about?" Sonny asked. Morgan filled her in. "That bastard Niles Kingman!" she grumbled. "What are you going to do about it?"

Morgan went back to the stove. The onions and garlic were soft. He turned off the heat, and checked his simmering stockpot.

"Morgan, I asked you what you were going to do about—"

"Nothing," he said.

"Nothing!" Sonny exploded.

"I'm not even going to let on to him that I know the truth," Morgan added.

"You mean you're just going to let him get away with it? Kingman *obviously* wanted to ruin your deal with Weiner so that you'd go into partnership with him!"

"Obviously," Morgan nodded. He took his pot of fish stock off the stove and carefully began to strain it through a colander lined with cheesecloth.

Sonny stamped her foot. "Morgan, how can you worry about cooking—" she paused, to sniff the air. "What *are* you cooking?"

"A sort of *zuppa di pesce*," he explained.

"It smells heavenly," she admitted. "But there's a time and a place, Morgan," she added, her anger once again beginning to snowball. "I mean, Niles Kingman has totally fucked you over!"

Morgan grinned. "You know what they say: sometimes it's best to just lie back and enjoy it."

"*What* has gotten *into* you!" she demanded angrily.

"Calm down and listen," he told her as he discarded the fish trimmings, transferred the strained stock back into the pot, and added the sauteed onion and garlic. "First of all, what's done is done. Weiner didn't offer to reinstate his deal with me." He put his chopped vegetables into the stockpot and put it back on the stove to bring it to a boil. "Secondly, if Weiner had offered to reinstate the deal, I wouldn't have accepted. To tell you the truth, the deal that Niles has offered DonSport is much better. By using already existing Kingman dealerships, our start-up costs are much less, which makes our break-even point much less, which means that our chance of success is much greater. And the fact that we don't have to build our own stores means that we can be in business on a nationwide scale that much sooner." He tasted the bubbling *zuppa*, added some pepper, a can of tomatoes, and a sliced-up lemon then turned it down to a simmer. "This'll cook for an hour or so. The fish goes in about twenty minutes before we're ready to eat."

"It just burns me up that Kingman thinks he's gotten away with a fast one," Sonny grumbled.

"Niles Kingman's meddling is the best thing that's happened to DonSport since 'Magnum P.I.' and 'Miami Vice' featured Ferraris." Morgan said. "Now, if you'll excuse me, I'd like to take a shower before we go watch the sunset."

That night she came to him. He'd been reading in bed, by candlelight, listening to the murmur of the bay coming in through the open windows. She tapped once on his bedroom door, then pushed it open, coming into the room and sitting down on the edge of the bed. Morgan put aside his book and looked at her. Her dark hair was down, and she was wearing that pale blue satin robe. She shrugged it off, not quite looking at him while she did it. She had nothing on underneath. In the candlelight, her supple skin was the hue of coffee with cream. Morgan threw back the covers, and she tucked herself in beside him. Not a word had been said. He drew the covers up over them both and began to kiss her. He was feeling dizzy; breathless with desire and passion for her.

She reached over to the nightstand to pinch out the candle flame, and then there was just the gentle sea breeze, and the starlight turning everything silvery blue.

Her limber, voluptuous body was intoxicating, and so very, wonderfully, different from the other women he'd known. Or maybe it was Sonny's *soul* that was different, or maybe *he* was different with Sonny, and why couldn't he think clearly enough to analyze this? And maybe *that* was what was different.

Then he stopped thinking. Oh, as always, Ilsa's ghost sought him out, but once he was inside Sonny, her warmth and embrace gave him shelter. He got a little frightened (old ghosts can be comforting in their familiarity), but Sonny was all around him like a silken veil, and he was molten; melded with her to make a perfect orb perpetually rolling through a silvery blue heaven.

This was love, Morgan thought. It had to be, and the only reason he doubted was because he had been so long without it that he'd forgotten how love felt. And then they were back on earth. Even Portofino seemed a pale comparison to where Morgan had been. They were breathing hard, sheened with perspiration, lying nestled in each other's arms.

"Wow," Sonny said. She rolled on top of him, her chin planted on his chest. "How was I?"

"What?"

"You heard me. How was I?"

"Now how did I know that you were going to ask something like that?" Morgan sighed. "Sonny, this isn't a race."

"I know it isn't a race. For one thing, it's how slow you can go, not how fast," she pointed out. "But I want to know if it was great for you, because it was great for me. *Really* great."

"It was great for me, too, Sonny."

She nodded confidently. "I thought so. I mean, why wouldn't it be?"

"Sonny," Morgan groaned. "You are making me crazy." He thought it over. "Or sane. I'm not sure which."

"But what I want to know is, was it . . . the best?"

He winked at her. "You fuck better than you make coffee, that's for sure."

"Morgan!" She waved a threatening fist under his nose.

"Okay." He rolled her off his chest and pinned her down. "But if you're so set on knowing if you're in first place, we're going to have to have another trial run."

She smiled smugly. "Okay by me, but you'll run out of gas before I do."

Morgan groaned. "These are lame jokes."

"I know." She buried her face against his chest. "But I don't know what to talk about right now," she said in confusion. "I'm more uptight now than I was before."

Her eyelashes tickled; her puffs of words were hot against his skin. Morgan thought: I won't look at her. I'll just stare up at the ceiling and listen. That way all I have to deal with is my pounding heart and the sound of her voice. "I don't know what to do or how to act, either," he confessed. "I'm glad this happened. I wanted it to happen. But now—"

"I know what you mean," she said quickly. "You need time to adjust to things. I understand that."

"I don't know what I mean," Morgan said truthfully. "You've got me all confused, Sonny." He grinned. "You've got me feeling like a teenager."

Her hand dipped down beneath the covers. Her fingers wrapped around him, and he began to swell. Sonny laughed triumphantly. "*I* think you feel like a teenager, as well."

"That's what I get for going to bed with Diana."

"Who?"

"Diana: Apollo's twin sister, daughter of Zeus and Leto."

"Are we talking about professional wrestling?"

"We're talking about the Lady of Wild Things; Huntswoman to the Gods." Morgan ran his hands down the curve of her spine to the swell of her bottom. "We're talking about you. Diana in a Burberry. Lady of the Speedway."

"You're making fun . . . Just because I'm . . . assertive." Sonny pretended to sulk. "I don't think you're being very nice at all."

"I'm about to remedy that," Morgan said. And he grabbed her.

Sonny woke up in Morgan's sun-filled bedroom wondering why she felt so different. It wasn't like she'd been a virgin before last night. She'd already been a woman, sexually experienced, knowing the score, and all that sort of garbage—

But now she felt like a woman, a *fulfilled* woman.

She reached out to touch him, gently, so as not to wake him up. The poor dear needed his sleep. He'd kept it up longer than she'd thought possible for any man in one night. But that probably had to do with the fact that he loved her, she thought happily. Of course, he probably didn't realize that, yet. Well, she wasn't going to tell him; let him figure it out on his own. She just wanted to run her hand over his body because he was finally beside her, and it had been one hell of a long haul to get him there.

She got out of bed and went to the window. The sun was so bright she had to shield her eyes against its reflection on the bay. It was a beautiful day, but then, she would have thought it was a beautiful day if she'd gone to the window and saw tornadoes and locusts and Nazis ripping through Portofino.

She went back to the bed, picked her robe up off the floor and balled it up, then put it beside Morgan's face. That way when he woke up, the first thing he'd smell would be her. She'd read about doing that to comfort puppies on their first night away from their mother, but she saw no reason why it shouldn't work with a man. She wanted to enchant Morgan. Oh, she was sure that deep down he loved her, but she knew enough about the world to understand that even *deep down, right* things can go wrong. Like what had happened between Morgan and her father. When Morgan had told her about it she'd been so hurt and angry, but she'd resolved it in her heart, and she'd forgiven Morgan. She wondered how long it would be before he could forgive himself.

She went into her own bedroom to get shorts and a T-shirt. She'd considered taking a shower, but she'd waited so long to make love to him that she wasn't about to wash his touch and taste and feel from her just yet. Downstairs on the first floor, she went out through the glass doors onto the terrace, and then down the old steps to the water's edge, her favorite spot in the whole villa. She sat down on the edge of the stone embankment and dangled her feet in the water. She thought about how it had been in bed with him. It'd been like driving at night on a deserted stretch of highway, when she'd closed her eyes for an instant, just to experience the scary exhilaration of hurtling along totally out of control for a second or two.

Except this had been so much better, because it lasted a lot longer than a couple of seconds, and she couldn't get hurt; well, at least she couldn't get killed.

Now all she had to do was get Morgan very used to making love with her. *"Make you my lovvve junkieee,"* she sang to herself, laughing out loud and kicking her feet in the water to make big splashes. It was going to be a dirty job, but somebody would have to do it. He'd said that he wanted some time to get used to things. That was fine with Sonny. She wanted him to have that time: to get used to the fact that he belonged to her.

She realized that she was to some degree being selfish about all this. She wanted him because she loved him; it was that simple. But she did have his best interests at heart as well. He loved her, after all, and he also needed her to help him in business. He was shrewd and sharp, but he showed too much mercy. Take this Niles Kingman thing. She saw Morgan's point about things working out to DonSport's advantage, but there was the principle of the matter to consider. Yeah, Morgan needed her; somebody more than willing, when the occasion warranted it, to kick a little ass.

All she needed were a couple more days with him all to herself. Lazy, hazy, barefoot days, keeping him drunk on the sun and the sea, and her body; keeping him from thinking, doubting, and questioning. A few more days and he'd belong to her.

And then she could take care of him, Sonny thought. The way he'd always taken care of her, she could care for him. They'd take care of each other. They really would be partners and equals, in bed and in the office. They'd be unstoppable. *Morgan and Thomas,* back together again, but in a very different way. And this time they'd be the perfect team.

"Sonny."

She turned to see him coming down the steps towards her, looking like a sexual fantasy in just his shorts and a day's growth of beard. He was grinning like a Goofy Gus. A shit-eating grin.

This is gonna be a piece of cake, Sonny gloated to herself. "You look happy," she told him.

"I am!"

I make you happy, Sonny thought, but did not say it to him. He'd have to figure it out for himself.

"I just got off the phone with Manfredi," he told her excitedly. "The Professor has put it all together for us. The race is on. I've telephoned a wire to Niles Kingman. We'll leave for Le Mans today."

Just a couple more days . . . "That's wonderful," Sonny brightly lied. "That's just perfect."

15

YOU'D THINK THAT *after you'd worked with a woman, and slept with her, you'd know her,* Morgan thought. Which goes to show that you don't know a damned thing.

The weirdness began as soon as they'd pulled out of Portofino. They'd put away their shorts and sneakers, put on their business clothes, and the weirdness began. Sonny's personality seemed to have changed; Morgan couldn't get a handle on it. If she'd been any colder during that eons-long, awkwardly silent car ride to the airport, Morgan would have turned on the Scorpio's heater.

It was nothing that Morgan could precisely put his finger on: Sonny was acting friendly, but in a remote and withdrawn manner; as untouchable as Eliot Ness. He left it alone all during the drive, but once they were settled on the flight to Paris he asked her what was going on. "Nothing," she said, and fixed him with a bright-eyed, vacant stare.

Morgan thought it over, and had an idea. "Sonny, is it on account of what happened between us last night?"

"What happened last night was terrific." Again, the simonized smile.

Morgan pushed up the armrests separating their seats and reached across to take her hand, but Sonny pulled away, lowering her armrest back into position. Pretty obvious symbolism there, he decided: *Road Closed.*

Sonny stared inquiringly. "Well?"

"Well what?" Morgan asked, smiling tentatively.

"Nothing. Nothing at all," she said, clenching her jaw. "Forget I said anything, okay?" And again she showed him that horrendous smile, rhinestone gaudy, and worth just about as much.

"Then why are you acting so weird?" Morgan tried one final time, although he was beginning to lose patience.

"Nothing's wrong," she repeated, but she said it like everything was wrong, and Morgan's heart began to ache, because beyond asking, he just didn't know what to do to make things better.

He tried to force the matter from his mind. He had work to do.

He wants to know what's wrong? Sonny thought icily. He's got the nerve to ask?

She glared at Morgan, who was busy jotting notes on a legal pad. He abruptly looked up at her and she turned on her smile like a flashlight. She just as quickly shut it off as he returned to his work.

What's wrong? she silently asked him. How about your *slam-bang-thank-you-ma'am* routine for sonofabitch starters?

But she wasn't going to say a word. Not one word. If he was going to get *so* preoccupied with business *so soon* after they'd become as *intimate* as it was *possible* for two people to *be*, then that was just *dandy* with her.

Hell, she was into business; she could be hard-edged and cold blooded . . . But not like the world's champion reptile seated beside her. She couldn't be so hard and cold as to put last night out of her mind (the way Mister *Iguana Heart* did) in the mad hurry-up to make this stupid flight to Paris.

He could have booked a later flight, just as a romantic gesture. After all that had happened between them the last couple of days he could have given her that much. The goddamned deal with that asshole Kingman wouldn't have fallen through if Morgan had booked a later flight.

In those few extra hours he could have swept her up in his arms, carried her to his bed, and made love to her one last time, or two, or three; not that it was the quantity that mattered as much as the *thought*. He might have *at least* taken her in his arms and told her that he *wanted* to make love to her again, but duty called—

And he might have said that he loved her. Or that he was at least thinking about loving her . . .

But he didn't do or say *any* of that. He just came halfway down those stone steps, told her that they were leaving for Le Mans, like she was his goddamned secretary, and then turned on his heel to hurry back up to the villa to pack.

And just now she'd given him another chance, and he'd blown it. She'd told him that she thought that last night had been terrific. She'd crawled out on a goddamned limb, and he hadn't picked up on it, hadn't mentioned last night at all. It was as if as far as he was concerned, last night was a pleasant memory.

Or had never happened?

Oh, shit. Sonny thought sadly. Was that the deal? Was she going to be right back where she started with this guy? She looked at Morgan, busy scribbling his notes. She could ask him, she supposed, but she knew that she'd never come right out and do that. Morgan would have to make the effort to *say*.

In fact, she'd done all she could do. The rest was up to him. He had to meet her at least a third of the way, and if he couldn't, then she would make do without him. She would still be a team player, giving him one hundred percent when it came to business. But when it came to love—

Well, Sonny Thomas would *die* for the man she loved. But she wouldn't crawl for *anybody*.

* * *

Paris, when they finally landed, was sunny, but with a brisk touch of fall in the air. As they exited from the terminal with their raincoats folded over their arms, and a redcap handling their luggage, they found that Nicole Houel had sent a limo for them. The driver took them directly to the La Défense quarter, where Nicole, in the gaudy tradition of P. T. Barnum, had called a news conference for the final day of the Paris Salon.

"Morgan, you look marvelous," Nicole exclaimed as she met them outside the stage door of the NCIT exhibition hall's auditorium. "So suntanned and healthy looking! Darling, you shall make a lovely magazine cover." She kissed him on the cheek, and in a stage-whisper clearly for Sonny's benefit, added, "I can't wait to see where the tan-line ends."

Sonny said murderously, "Morgan, isn't this *Nile Kingman*'s friend?"

"And whose little girl are you?" Nicole calmly regarded Sonny.

Morgan introduced the two women to each other as Nicole stepped in close and tried to establish property rights by fussing with his tie. Sonny and Nicole were being barely civil to one another, acting the way Sylvester the Cat and Tweety-Bird do when Grannie's around. Morgan had this image of him turning his back and then the pickaxes would come out.

But he just couldn't deal with Lady Wrestlemania right now. He was too busy trying not to toss his cookies due to an awful case of stage fright over the imminent press conference. He stepped out on stage as far as the wing to peek around at the crowd.

The *large* crowd.

The *very* large crowd.

The "Viewpoint" interview had been a relatively private affair: just himself, the interviewer, and the camera team. It'd been a very long time since Morgan had stood up before this many people.

He heard the two women coming up behind him. Nicole explained that in addition to the representatives from the automotive press and Parisian media, she'd seen to it that the wire services and several freelance film teams were present to feed the stateside news organizations and the sports-oriented cable networks. She'd also prepared and distributed a press kit covering the basic details of the race, and just enough about the DonSport, America concept to ensure it's prominence in the resulting media coverage.

"Whenever you're ready," Nicole told Morgan. "Just look at me and nod when you want to cue me to end it."

He felt a firm hand pushing against the small of his back and turned to see Sonny smiling at him. Thank goodness it was a real smile. "Those magazine covers are hanging around empty, just waiting for you," she winked. "Knock 'em dead, boss."

Morgan nodded, swallowed, and stepped out before the murmuring audience. The murmuring ceased, and all he could hear was his pounding heart. He hated it when he was still yards from the mike, and the crowd was quiet and attentive and watching him walk. And then he was up against a colorful backdrop featuring the various carmakers' marques, swarming like a fighter escort around the huge, emblazoned *DonSport, America*. The backdrop was splendid, and as he tried to be suitably photogenic while the flashbulbs popped, he made a mental note to compliment Nicole. She was turning out to be a first rate publicist.

He made the short speech he'd written during the plane ride: he announced his business's expansion, the kickoff Le Mans event, and the subsequent American tour of the participating cars.

Then it was time for questions:

"Hey, Don, who will you be driving for?"

"Why, DeManto of course. As some of you may be old enough to remember, I've had occasion to learn their gearshift pattern."

There were a few appreciative chuckles. He began to loosen up.

"What's the significance of the race?"

"You mean beyond us having a good time and giving all of you something to write about?" More laughter. As it subsided, he waited a few beats, and then launched into his rap. "Seriously, anyone interested in cars, and driving, has a strong opinion concerning the merits and weaknesses of various high-performance automobiles. This race should, in large measure, put an end to that controversy, thanks to the willingness of those manufacturers who have accepted our challenge to put their vehicles—and their reputations—on the line. In three days that sizable part of the public that looks at cars as more than just a means of getting from here to there, is going to find out just which cars are the best, within their engine classes, of course. The average race merely answers the question of which *racing* car is king of the *track*. This race is going to answer the question of which *street legal* car is *king of the road.*"

There were several other questions concerning practical matters about the race, and then Morgan got nailed by the query he'd been dreading, and knew would eventually come:

"How does it feel to be returning to Le Mans?"

He hesitated. The usual quotable, if trite phrases had long since sprung to mind: "It's glorious, *magnifique!* Words fail me! blah-blah-blah."

Morgan was about to utter them. What was the point of bringing everyone down by reminding them that he'd walked away from racing due to the Le Mans event in which Lee Thomas died? This was a lightweight, promotional press conference; there was no point in playing that sad song—

Then Morgan caught a glimpse of Sonny watching from the wings, and it dawned on him that maybe the reason she was being so moody had to do with the fact that he'd made tremendous demands on her, but left her out of all the glory. It made sense. He knew that all this commotion over the race was merely hype, but he'd been through it before. She hadn't. She was just a kid.

Yes, she really was just a kid, the thought echoed, making him feel guilty all over again about taking her to bed, and for taking her as someone of his own generation, with his own values and outlook on life.

On the other hand, they'd been damn good in bed . . . The conflicting thoughts and feelings whirled inside his head and heart. He thought he might be in love with Sonny, but he knew from past, bitter experience that love was often not enough . . . Sonny seemed to love him, when she wasn't being angry . . .

Morgan snapped out of his reverie; the auditorium was waiting for an answer. He could sort out his personal quandaries another time. Right now, he was fairly certain that the reason Sonny was displeased with him was because she was feeling cheated: she wanted a little piece of the limelight. Morgan was going to see that she got it.

"I'm made very sad by the idea of returning to Le Mans," Morgan began softly.

His sudden, downbeat tone and unexpected words sent a murmuring ripple through the audience of reporters and camera people. Out of the corner of his eye he saw Nicole Houel's warning frown. He ignored it.

"I want to say a few words about a past racing great. A man named Lee Thomas. Many of you here are too young to have seen Lee Thomas drive, but if you have any love at all for the sport of Grand Prix, you should make it a point to be familiar with Lee Thomas' brilliant career. He was my mentor, and we drove together on the same team a lot." Morgan fixed his gaze on the auditorium's far wall. He didn't want to get distracted, or lose his chain of thought. It was essential to Sonny, to himself, and to Lee's memory that he got this right. "As some of you may remember, I was on Lee's BXI team when he lost his life at Le Mans. When Lee died, I quit racing to begin DonSport, the success of which we're here to celebrate today. Lee was a part of DonSport in its conception, and his spirit remains at DonSport, in part, thanks to his daughter Sonny Thomas, a terrific driver in her own right, and an executive in my organization." Morgan looked at her standing in the wings. "Sonny, come on out."

He watched her frantically shake her head in horror, refusing to come on stage, but Morgan waited stubbornly, and finally she ducked out of the wings and into the cameras' bright lights, where she looked adorable and demure. "Sonny Thomas has been appointed a vice president at DonSport, in charge of administering our expansion effort. I suspect you'll want to interview her at some point on the specifics of how DonSport, America is going to work."

Sonny gracefully made her exit back into the wings, whereupon she simultaneously stuck out her tongue, gave Morgan the finger, and then stalked off, disappearing from his view. Morgan grinned and turned back to face the audience.

"Getting back to the original question, I want you all to know that as far as I'm concerned this race is dedicated with love and respect to one of racing's legends, Lee Thomas." He nodded, more to himself than to the audience. "I think you'll all understand just how serious I *am* about honoring Lee, when the race is finished."

Some of the reporters tried to follow up on his last mysterious comment, but Morgan glanced at Nicole and nodded, and she hurried out.

"I afraid that's all the questions we have time for, right now," Nicole announced as Morgan made a hasty retreat. He heard Nicole promise that he would be available for more interviews at Le Mans; that the cars would go directly from the race to America, to begin the tour of the Kingman and Son dealerships where DonSport, America outlets were to open. As Morgan went in search of Sonny he heard Nicole add that Niles Kingman and his father were already in Le Mans to orchestrate matters from that end, arranging for the use of the circuit and booking blocks of hotel rooms for the drivers, works teams, and journalists converging on the town. The flat-bed transports were already hauling the cars to the Sarthe Valley. She reiterated that for the convenience of the media, which had congregated to cover the Paris Salon, the race would be held in three days; a schedule designed to give everyone involved a chance to arrive, fiddle with their cars, and get a day's rest before the event.

And to give the hotels and restaurants of Le Mans a chance to make a decent profit, Morgan added to himself.

Nicole added that drivers could take practice runs around the circuit if they wished, but as this was an unofficial race, there would be no preliminary qualifying runs. Starting positions would go according to engine size: fastest cars up front.

Several of the participating car manufacturers' P.R. people then took turns at the microphone praising DonSport and making confident predictions about the race's outcome, when Morgan found Sonny waiting outside the auditorium.

"Everything okay between us, now?" he asked hopefully.

"What?"

"You're not angry anymore, right? I mean, the fact that you weren't getting your fair share of the credit for all of this *was* the reason you were upset?"

"You mean that's what all that 'bring the little lady out and give her a big hand' bullshit was all about?" She started to laugh. "I don't know about you, Morgan." Her laughter trailed off. "I don't know about us." She shook her head. "What am I going to do with you?"

"Well," Morgan smiled, "You could do more of what you did with me last night in Portofino—"

She put her finger to his lips. "Is that what *you want*,

Morgan? Or is it what you think *I* want? Or is it what you think you're supposed to *say?*"

"Dammit, Sonny!" He took several steps away and then turned back to face her. "All I was trying to do was flirt. Just have a little fun." He scowled, looking away. "I don't know. We seem to be out of synch. Instead of it getting easier between us it's getting harder."

She nodded, looking rueful. "And it's not all your fault, is that what you're thinking but not saying?"

"Maybe it is," he agreed quietly.

"But it was nice the way you brought my father into it, and you *were* thinking of me when you made that announcement giving me credit." She began to smile. "I guess it was *kind* of a romantic gesture on your part, hmm?"

"What are we talking about now?" Morgan asked hopelessly.

"Us . . . life . . . love," Sonny whimsically replied, and then grew serious. "I know I'm not easy to please." She put her arms around his neck and began to kiss him lightly on the mouth. "But I'm worth it."

Morgan slid his hands down to her waist and began returning her kisses. He had no idea what had just happened, but she wasn't acting weird anymore; at least, she wasn't acting unpleasantly weird, so thank heaven for small favors. For the next few days he expected to be spending most of his time running around putting out small fires. If he'd managed to placate Sonny for the moment that was terrific. A nice Sonny Thomas was a very nice thing, indeed. And it meant he could get on with the other business at hand.

Sonny abruptly pulled away. "We'll continue this later." She ran her hands down her sides to smooth her clothes. "Here comes Brigitte Bardot."

Morgan turned to see Nicole approaching. "It is three thirty!" she admonished, her accent thickening, as Morgan had noticed it did whenever she got excited.

"You two must get on the road, or you will be caught in the rush traffic leaving Paris! In Le Mans we all have rooms at the Provence—"

"No," Morgan said. "I never stay in a chain hotel.

"Morgan!" Nicole complained. "It is *très chic!*"

"Usually when I was at Le Mans I stayed at the Ricordeau, in Loué," Morgan said.

"Oh, but you cannot!" Nicole rolled her eyes. "It is almost thirty kilometers from Le Mans! I need you close at hand, darling! For the press—"

"And there's so much business to attend to," Sonny softly reminded him. "I hate to admit it, but this time she's right."

Morgan nodded wearily. "Okay. But I still won't stay at a chain hotel, no matter how chic it thinks it is," he declared. "I'll book Sonny and me into rooms at the Alexandra," he told Nicole. "It borders on the Plaza de la République. You can't get more in-town than that." He winked at Sonny. "You'll like it. It'll be a welcome dose of sensory excess after laid-back Portofino, and we'll be close to the old quarter of the town, which is really the nicest part of Le Mans."

Nicole shook her head. "You'll never get a reservation at this late date."

Morgan just smiled. "One thing the good innkeepers of Le Mans understand is that if the race car drivers aren't happy, *nobody* is going to be happy. Hold our reservations at the Provence, you'll be needing them for the reporters about to be bumped out of the Alexandra on our behalf. I'll phone from here, and then we'll get on the road. By the way, how are you getting there?"

"I rented a car," Nicole replied.

"That's a relief," Sonny whispered to Morgan.

If Nicole heard the remark, she didn't let on. "I'll be leaving as soon as I'm done here. Niles and his father would like us three to have dinner with them." She paused. "You don't mind *eating* in a chain hotel, do you, darling?"

* * *

Morgan and Sonny left Paris at four that afternoon, driving a DeManto Gatto, the limited edition, turbo-charged, four wheel drive car which was to be the company's entry in the race.

The traffic quickly thinned once they were out of Paris, and heading southwest on A11, via Chartres, into the Loire region. Morgan and Sonny took turns driving and had a great time putting the red convertible through its tire squealing, turboshrill paces. Morgan wasn't especially worried about conserving the car. Professor DeManto was taking no chances: an experienced support team, a trailer full of spare parts, *and* a spare Gatto were all waiting at Le Mans.

As they entered the Sarthe Valley, Morgan remembered that years ago one of the first things he'd noticed about the region was that the buildings here were all constructed of stone. He'd asked Lee Thomas about it.

"Boyo," Thomas had grinned. "The stone says that these people believe in permanence. They fought the Romans, followed Joan of Arc, and endured the Nazis. They know that governments and leaders come and go, but that they will always have their blue sky, green pastures, their wide, calm rivers, and their vineyards. Building in stone was their way of making their homes permanent, too. So the upper classes erected grand châteaux and castles on the sweat and labor of honest working people." Lee Thomas had winked at Morgan. "And these good, shrewd, normally dour people know one other thing: that for as long as there are motor cars, and men to drive them, once a year they can let their hair down and indulge in the excitement of their 24 Heurs du Mans."

As Lee's apprentice, Morgan quickly learned that "excitement" was hardly the word for the frenzy that descended upon Le Mans in advance of its famous 24 hour race. Today, as they approached the turn-off for

Le Mans they received an omen that the good people of the region were more than ready to get it up for his own publicity race. A motorcycle cop on the A11 intercepted the Gatto, intending to pull them over for the speeding ticket that they richly deserved. But the cop evidently recognized Morgan, and not only waved them on, he also escorted them, red lights flashing, siren wailing, for the last few miles of fast lane before the Le Mans exit, to keep the mere mortals out of their regal path.

That was how far and fast word of the race had traveled. That was the power of Le Mans.

They arrived at their destination just two hours after leaving Paris. It was dark as Morgan drove directly to the Le Mans racing circuit just south of the town. He pulled into the flood-lit paddocks, where the flatbed haulers and parts trailers were parked, to check in with Fabiano Manfredi who was heading up the DeManto works team. Fabi, looking quite like a WW II commando in his matching black wool slacks, heavy turtleneck, and wool knit watch cap, and with that magnificent handlebar moustache of his was wildly gesticulating orders to his people as Morgan pulled up.

Fabi took away the Gatto, apologizing, but explaining to Morgan that it wouldn't do to risk the two hundred thousand dollar thoroughbred machine in the stop and go traffic of the city, just 72 hours before the big race.

As Morgan handed over the keys and unloaded his and Sonny's luggage from the car's trunk, he noticed several mammoth vehicle transport trucks, with "Kingman and Son" painted on the sides of their cab's doors, parked along the edge of the paddock area. A half-dozen men were loitering around the trucks, smoking cigarettes and passing around a bottle.

Manfredi saw Morgan looking that way. "Do not bother going over and talking to them, Donaldo. I tried and almost had my head chopped off for my trouble."

Morgan turned around. "I don't get it?"

"Neither do I, my friend," Manfredi shrugged. "They are all English fellows. I wished to discuss with them the arrangements for transporting the race cars to America, but—" he hesitated.

"But what, Fabi?"

He shook his head. "Oh, forget that I said anything. Perhaps I was too brusque with them. I do grow short-tempered, and my nerves always run away with me before a race."

Manfredi handed over the keys to a pair of run-of-the-mill, ninety grand, white DeManto coupés, which would just have to do as their basic transportation around town. Sonny followed Morgan back to Le Mans to check into their hotel. Built in the Renaissance style, with arched doorways, interior friezes of cherubs and satyrs, and a showplace lobby with a magnificent coffered ceiling, the Alexandra was once the residence of a deputy of Louis XIII. As Morgan had explained to Sonny, the Alexandra was firmly entrenched as a class act hotel, even if it had grown a little seedy around the edges; the Vieux Mans, Le Man's medieval quarter on the banks of the Sarthe, with its stepped alleys and winding streets, its boutiques and restaurants, was just a stone's throw away, so the location more than made up for the hotel's occasional bit of cracked plaster or threadbare patch of carpeting.

The front desk staff seemed to be in genuine anguish over the fact that they had been unable to find Morgan and Sonny adjoining rooms. Morgan would have taken their crocodile tears more seriously if the hotel hadn't also put them on separate floors, but he was too exhausted to argue. They just had time to unpack, shower, and change before meeting Nicole and the Kingmans for dinner.

Morgan put on a dark gray suit and went down to the lobby to meet Sonny. She wore a flowing, gray and white patterned dress with a plunging, lace inset bodice. As he watched her move across the hotel's busy lobby to meet him he took pleasure in the fact that

Sonny was turning heads now just as she had in Paris, and everywhere else she went.

Sonny drove them the short distance to the Provence, on the Ave du Gal-Leclerc, near the twin towered Abbey of la Couture. They turned the car over to a parking valet and went into the glitzy lobby, with its abundance of chrome, smoked glass, and hissing fountains that reminded Morgan of New York's Trump Tower arcade. They found the restaurant, where Nicole and Niles and Sam Kingman were already seated near yet another splashing fountain.

"I should have worn a wet suit," Sonny murmured as the tuxedoed maître d' led them to the table.

Niles and his father, framed by silver champagne buckets, stood up as Morgan and Sonny approached.

Niles was dressed in some kind of modified cowboy suit. In addition to his cordovan high-heeled boots, he was wearing silver arrowheads on the points of his shirt collar, one of those odd, shoestring ties held at his throat by a silver clasp, and a maroon suit with contrasting silver stitching on the lapels and pocket flaps.

"Do you think he asked the valet to park his horse?" Sonny whispered to Morgan.

Sam Kingman was in his early seventies. He was big bellied, and maybe five and a half feet tall. He had his son's florid coloring and red hair, although most of the latter had long since disappeared except for a horseshoe wreath around his head. He was dressed conservatively in dark blue, Brooks Brothers 346.

He was wearing a diamond pinkie ring big enough to choke a horse.

"Long time, Don, right, kiddo?" Sam said, extending his hand.

"Long time, Sam," Morgan agreed, shaking hands. Meanwhile he was smiling at Nicole who was seated at the table and trying hard not to be too obvious about staring down her cleavage. *Her* low-cut black dress made Sonny's lace bodice look like a turtleneck.

216

Sonny cleared her throat. It figured that she'd be the one to notice him staring. She managed to give him a kick in the shin that brought tears to his eyes but went unnoticed by the others.

"May I introduce Sonny Thomas," Morgan said through clenched teeth. "Sonny, this is Sam Kingman," he glared at her. "And I believe you know everyone else."

"Oh yes," Sonny said sweetly. "I've meet Ms. Houel, and then there's dear Niles . . . Didn't I run into you at a party given by Weiner, Carlson, and—"

"If you'll excuse us for one second," Morgan hastily cut her off. He grabbed her elbow to drag her away from the table, and when he was sure they were out of earshot he hissed, "How would you like to be murdered?"

"And what about the race?" she shot back. "If I'm murdered, I can't drive." She maneuvered him so that his back was to the table and then gently but firmly squeezed his crotch. "Keep your eyes where they belong and your mind on business, fella. At *your* age a man better save his dwindling strength for the *real* thing."

As she returned to the table, Sam Kingman hurried to pull out her chair for her. "A little business conference," she explained in reply to the curious stares.

"Miss Thomas," Sam grinned, "Allow me to pour you some champagne. You know, I met your daddy once. Quite a man, Lee Thomas was. I understand you're following in his footsteps."

"I'm trying to, Mister Kingman."

"Good, good," Sam Kingman nodded. "Sonny, I had this idea for a promotion; I was just talking to Nicole and Niles about it. You know, women account for a sizable portion of automobile sales, these days. I see a series of TV commercials with you offering driving tips to the women . . . They would be sort of like the kind Jackie Stewart gives for Ford, except your tips would exploit the feminine angle, you know?"

"Nothing too aggressive, right?" Sonny asked with a straight face.

"Right!" Sam Kingman nodded enthusiastically. "Oh, and you'd drive different cars in each commercial, see? The idea would be to build customer loyalty to Kingman and Son dealerships, not to any one make of car, you know?"

"I think that's a marvelous idea," Sonny said diplomatically, patting Sam's hand. "But first things, first, Mr. Kingman. We've got a lot of business to discuss concerning the events about to take place right now, right here in Le Mans . . ."

Sam Kingman laughed. "Okay, honey . . . She's sharp . . ." he nodded sagely to the table in general. "Don," he said, making a big production out of winking, "maybe you want to sell her to me, what do you say, kiddo?"

"I think I'd better hang on to her, Sam," Morgan said mildly.

"Another marvelous idea," Sonny quietly murmured, eyeing Morgan.

"Everybody be sure to order an appetizer," Sam was loudly instructing the table. "What they call dinner in these *nouvelle* joints wouldn't feed a bird."

The meal, and then the business discussions over coffee, dragged on. It'd been a long day, with a lot of traveling for both of them. Morgan could see that Sonny was fading fast. "Why don't you go back to the hotel and get a good night's sleep?" he suggested to her during a lull in the conversation.

Sonny, trying to stifle a yawn, shot a worried glance at Nicole, who looked bright eyed and wide awake. "But Morgan, I drove us here. How will you get back to the hotel?"

"Oh, don't worry," Nicole smiled at her. "I will take care of him." She paused for an evil beat. "I mean, I will see that he—"

"I *know* what you mean, Ms. Houel," Sonny replied evenly. "But I *am* exhausted. So, if you'll all excuse me . . ." As the men got up, Sonny took the opportunity to whisper in Morgan's ear, "Come to my room when you get back to the hotel."

"If it's not too late," Morgan whispered back, but he wasn't sure that Sonny had heard him in the flurry of "good-nights" being exchanged. And then she was gone.

The discussion continued for another half hour. At one point Nicole excused herself, and a minute or so later, Niles left the table.

When they were alone, Sam Kingman, who was puffing on a foot-long cigar, winked at Morgan. "I think my boy has a hankering for that little French lady."

"He has good taste," Morgan said. In women, if not in clothes, he thought to himself.

"In women, if not in clothes," Sam Kingman said, busy shaping the ash on the tip of his cigar against the ashtray's lip. "You know, I'm very pleased with this deal Niles has put together with you. I think it's going to be profitable for all concerned."

"I certainly expect it to be, Sam."

"You know, it's real different from anything we've been into before," Sam elaborated, fixing Morgan with a level gaze. "It's requiring us to expand certain aspects of our business. Like our European and stateside transport operation." He paused. "Morgan, let me ask you something. You know your way around Europe. In England is it usual for honest working men to be . . . well . . . *tough?*"

"I'm not sure I know what you're getting at, Sam."

"Well, take those guys crewing our trucks over by the race track. I was over there with Niles, earlier, you know, and I went over to talk to those guys. Now, I figure I'm a pretty good judge of character." He grinned at Morgan. "You got to be when you sell cars, or sell anything, for a living. Anyways, I go over to those guys manning our trucks, and what I see is a bunch of punks, you know? Real garbage. And they

were uppity to *me,* even *after* I told them who I am."
He scowled at his cigar. "And they didn't seem to know
shit about the transport business." Sam shrugged, and
then looked around, as if to make sure no one could
overhear him. "And there was one last thing. While I
was standing there, one of 'em bent over to pick up
something, and his jacket rode up, and Don, I'm pretty
sure I saw a gun sticking up out of his pants, right back
there in the small of his back, you know?"

Morgan nodded. He thought about Fabiano
Manfredi's misgivings about the men, but he decided
not to mention it to Sam. All he needed now was for
the elder Kingman to get cold feet and quash the entire
deal. "Well, it could've been a legally owned gun,"
Morgan mused. "Maybe he had it to protect the truck
and its cargo from being hijacked. But if you're concerned about it, Sam, why don't you ask Niles?"

"Nah," Sam blushed, and then shrugged. "I mean,
what's the big deal? Anyways, I'll be honest with you,
kiddo. At present, I'm not interested in rocking the
boat with my son. It's no big secret him and me haven't
been getting along too well, up until this deal with you
came about, that is. I owe you one for that," he smiled
gratefully. "Anyways, if I questioned Niles about these
new men he's hired . . . Well, you know . . . he might
take it the wrong way, think I'm trying to take over this
baby or looking to find fault with him like he claims I
always do." He made a gesture of dismissal with his
cigar. "Here they come back. Now don't say anything
about any of this nonsense. Besides, maybe I'm just a
picky old man, but when you get to be my age, kiddo,
you'll find yourself acting just the same way."

Sam laughed, but his eyes revealed his concern.

It was two in the morning by the time Morgan
managed to get himself back to the Alexandra, with
Nicole's lengthy list of his appointments for tomorrow
folded in his pocket. He'd politely refused Nicole's
invitation to bunk with her, and even her offer of a

ride. It was a pleasant night, and Morgan thought a brisk walk the short distance back to his hotel might serve to quiet his still buzzing mind.

Back at the hotel, when the elevator operator asked him what floor, Morgan hesitated. Sonny had more or less commanded a performance, but he'd been up eighteen hours, and logged a hell of a lot of miles of travel. What he wanted most was a comfortable bed and sleep. He would have been very happy to have Sonny cuddled up beside him as his teddy bear, but tonight, cuddling was *all* he was up for. He had a feeling she wouldn't understand. Better to go to his own room, he decided, and relayed his floor number to the elevator operator.

Once there he undressed quickly and flopped into bed. He phoned down for an eight o'clock wake-up call and clicked off the bedside lamp. He thought sadly that it was likely that Sonny was going to be pissed off with him tomorrow, but he was so tired that not even that troubling thought was enough to keep him from dropping off into a deep sleep.

16

THE WAKE-UP CALL jolted Morgan out of a vivid dream: he had left his bride-to-be Ilsa Wolff waiting at the altar, because he was too drunk to find the church. At some point, Ilsa became Sonny, and while he was staggering around, trying to make Nicole Houel understand where she was to drive him, he heard over a radio that Sonny had been killed in a car crash.

The dream's antecedents were obvious, but that didn't make it any less unsettling, seeing that Sonny would be driving the race for him day after tomorrow. Morgan, lying in bed and staring up at the ceiling, felt smothered by an intense wave of dread. He had the strongest urge to call everything off.

He took a long, hot shower, and then had breakfast in his room. By his third cup of coffee, the impact of the dream was fading, and he was starting to feel human again. He phoned Sonny's room, but there was no answer. He called down to the desk to see if she'd left the hotel, and found that she had.

He checked Nicole's list: his first meeting was scheduled to begin in a half hour at the racing circuit. He called downstairs to have his car brought around, pulled a sports jacket on over his turtleneck sweater, and went out to do battle with the world.

As Morgan drove into the circuit pit area he saw Sonny talking with some reporters near the DeManto works. She looked relaxed and self-assured handling herself with the press. She was wearing faded blue jeans, a bulky red and purple swirled sweater that he guessed was a Missoni, and black Reeboks. Watching her, taking pleasure in watching her, Morgan thought that she looked like she belonged in the public eye.

He waited until she was free and then went over. As he'd guessed last night, she was not happy to see him.

"I waited up for you" were the first words to come out of her mouth.

"Sonny, the meeting with Niles and Sam dragged on forever. By the time I got back to the hotel I was exhausted."

"Nicole drive you back?" Sonny asked, her voice tight.

"No, she didn't, as a matter of fact—"

"Oh?" she cut him off. "Maybe you didn't *come* back," she snapped. "Maybe your meeting dragged on so long it was more convenient for you to go up to *her* hotel room—"

Morgan lost it. He just blew his top. He restrained the urge to shake some sense into her, but before he quite knew what he was doing, he said, "I slept by myself last night, but if I *want* to sleep with Nicole or *any* woman, I'll do it, and I don't have to ask permission from a spoiled brat like you—"

"Is that what I am to you, Morgan? A brat?"

"You are right now, Sonny," Morgan said flatly. "Look, I've got to meet some people. I'll see you later."

But that was the last Morgan saw of Sonny that day.

Sonny watched Morgan stomp off. She stifled her urge to call him back and apologize. It would do him good to let him chew on the fact that she was feeling angry. He'd been taking her for granted.

But as soon as he was out of sight, she started rationalizing. Hell, she could see that from his point of view, he'd probably think that *she*'d been taking *him* for granted. And maybe she *had* been a *trifle* bratty . . .

And it was a good bet that old Nicole with the laugh lines around her eyes would be shrewd enough not to greet Morgan first thing with a frown and a complaint.

Oh, shit, Sonny thought to herself. Now that *she'd* cooled off, it occurred to her that if she wanted to win Morgan she had to start thinking strategy.

The problem gnawed at her all morning. To make matters worse, she didn't happen to run into Morgan, so she couldn't apologize or give him the chance to apologize to her, which would have been even better . . .

She had a lunch appointment with an AP correspondent at a grill in the old quarter, near the hotel. As she passed through the dark restaurant's crowded bar she happened to see Niles Kingman—he was pretty hard to miss; there weren't too many cowboy hats in Le Mans—having a drink with another man. Niles was laughing and talking loudly; Sonny, eavesdropping, heard him bragging about sleeping with Nicole last night . . .

She managed to get past Niles without him seeing her. As she sat down at the AP correspondent's table she felt miserable over doubting Morgan. She had, of course, believed him when he'd told her that he'd slept alone; it was just that now she believed him a little more than she had previously. Morgan was right about one other thing: she *had* been an awful, shrewish brat to have sent him away angry this morning.

All through lunch she had a hard time keeping her mind on the interview. She couldn't wait to hightail it back to the hotel on the off chance that Morgan would be there. He wasn't, of course, and none of the numerous messages waiting for her were from him.

He was probably still sulking over the morning's quarrel, she thought to herself, and found that she was kind of pleased at the idea. It stood to reason that a woman couldn't make a guy miserable unless he cared a lot about her.

Oh well, the more miserable Morgan was now, the

sweeter their reconciliation would be tonight. She quickly jotted him a note *(I'm so sorry!/XXXXX til tonight/Yer Brat/S)*, left it for him at the front desk, and got as far as the door, when she reconsidered. The note was kind of icky and juvenile, and he probably already thought she was enough of a child . . . She went back and retrieved the note, crumbled it, and threw it away. It'd be better to surprise Morgan tonight.

That's what she'd do. Just show up at his room, take him to bed, and prove to him first hand just how sorry she was for doubting him.

Morgan got back to his hotel about nine, after having a quick dinner with some people from the ESPN satellite sports network who'd flown over to cover the race. He knew some of the reporters from back when he'd had his own ill-fated stint as a TV commentator, and rehashing old times had been fun, but he couldn't totally relax: the bad vibes from the fight he'd had with Sonny that morning were still with him. Actually, they'd intensified as the day went on. He'd handled the situation badly, he now realized. If he was so much older and wiser than Sonny, he was going to have to use some of that wisdom in dealing with her.

If only she weren't so intense, Morgan thought as he rode the elevator up to his floor. But then Sonny— wherever she'd disappeared to all day—was probably wondering why he had to be so mellow.

When Morgan opened the door to his hotel room he saw Nicole Houel in his bed, the covers pulled up to her neck, her curly red hair fanned out against the pillows.

"How did you get in here?" he demanded.

"I showed the maid my press pass and told her that I was supposed to meet you here. She let me in with her key. I tried to give her a tip, but she wouldn't accept it. It seems the entire town cannot do enough for anyone connected with this race of yours."

"Well, that was very sneaky," Morgan said.

"Yes," she sighed theatrically. "I *am* very sneaky."

"And just what kind of meeting did you have in mind?"

"Oh, do not torture me!" she admonished, her accent thickening delightfully as the words cascaded from her pouting lips. "We will discuss business later, but now I want to play!" She looked at him questioningly. "Aren't you glad I'm here?"

Morgan thought it over. So sue me, he decided. "Yeah, I guess I am," he wearily admitted. He tossed his keys onto the bureau, then took off his jacket and hung it on the back of a chair. "Right now, I *need* someone to play with."

"It is Sonny who has made you feel so sad, yes?"

Morgan looked at her and nodded.

Nicole cocked her head. "Has she made you feel old?"

Morgan blushed.

"*C'est dommage.*" She threw back the covers. She was nude, and Morgan, looking at her, felt himself stiffening. The wafting blankets sent him the dizzying scent of her own sexual excitement.

She smiled and patted the bed. "Come to me, darling. I will show you that what you need is a woman, not a fickle child."

He undressed quickly, and slid into bed beside her. He tried to lose himself in her kisses, and the fragrant, silky weight of her breasts, but what he felt as he entered her, moving in rhythm with her supple hips, was not passion, but safety. With Nicole, he realized, he could have physical release and intense, exquisite pleasure without the danger of suffering an equally intense, exquisite misery. As Nicole cried out in the throes of her climax, and as Morgan felt his own, shivery spasms begin to rise along his spine, he thought of Sonny, and hoped that she could someday forgive him. But he just didn't want to risk his heart anymore.

Afterward, as Morgan lay quietly, staring up at the ceiling, Nicole cuddled him, sighing happily. "You have become quite an addiction with me, you know."

"That's nice to hear," Morgan said, and tried to sound convincing.

Nicole rose up on one elbow to look at him. "Why so moody?" she asked softly.

Morgan forced a smile. "I'm sorry." There was no way he was going to talk about Sonny, so he lied. "I guess I'm just a little preoccupied with business, and the race."

"And that is only natural," Nicole declared. She got out of bed to fetch her cigarettes from her purse. "And if our play is done, then we should discuss business. Darling, considering what we mean to each other, surely you can now tell me when and where the truck will arrive?"

Morgan watched her light a cigarette, and then cross the room to the desk, where she dropped the spent match into an ashtray. "What truck are you talking about?"

"Morgan!" she scolded, cutting him off. "There is no longer any need to be coy with me. We shall be working—and, hopefully, *playing* together—for a long time to come." She shook her head, chuckling. "You and Niles are so into your silly, little cloak-and-dagger games."

"Nicole, what's in that cigarette you're smoking?"

"Morgan, you must stop these games before you make me angry," she frowned. "I've been very patient with both you and Niles, but the time has come to realize that we are all equal partners in this endeavor."

"Look, now I'm the one beginning to lose patience. Will you please tell me what you're talking about?"

"You know very well what I am talking about!" she insisted. "The whereabouts of that tractor-trailer full of stolen art that you and Niles and I will be smuggling into America!"

"What?" Morgan jackknifed up out of the bed. "What is going on?" he demanded angrily.

Nicole, standing with one hand resting on her cocked hip, took a long drag of her cigarette and scrutinized him with narrowed eyes. "I'm talking about a fortune in stolen art. Artwork that we will hide in the automobiles to be sent to America for the publicity tour." She smiled. "You seem at a loss for words, darling? Did you and Niles really think I was going to believe that story he fed me about your being an innocent dupe?"

Morgan sat on the edge of the bed and rested his head in his hands. "It's starting to make sense to me, now," He looked up at Nicole and frowned. "I'm an innocent dupe, all right." He clenched his fists in frustration. "Make that innocent *dope!* Everything is finally beginning to make sense. Dammit! All this time that phony cowboy has had me jumping through hoops like a trained dog. I had a legitimate deal going with a San Francisco venture capital firm—"

"Yes, of course," she said impatiently. "Weiner, Carlson and Boyd."

"How do *you* know about that?"

"Niles told me all about it, of course. He'd gone to them to try and borrow money—"

"Why the hell would Niles Kingman need to borrow money?"

"Darling, you really must stop this foolish charade," she warned, watching him carefully.

"Nicole, please," Morgan held out his hands. "Please, just humor me. Pretend that I don't know what we're talking about and start from the beginning."

Nicole, stubbing out her cigarette, suddenly smiled. "My God, you really *don't* know, do you?"

"That's what I've been *telling* you," Morgan sighed.

She began to laugh. "Oh, Morgan, it is too funny," she shook her head as she went to the bed and sat down beside him, resting her hand on his knee. "It is a good thing I'm fond of you darling. You're going to need me to take care of you from now on."

"Just tell me what's going on," Morgan gruffly demanded. "From the beginning, please."

"Certainly," she said, amused. "It began in London,

where Niles Kingman had run up tremendous losses at a private, after-hours gambling club run by organized crime. If you remember, I mentioned that to you some time ago. What was worse for poor Niles, he'd gambled away funds he'd borrowed from one of London's toughest loan sharks in order to buy stolen art."

"Hold it, you're starting to lose me again," Morgan complained.

"That's why Niles was in London in the first place, darling. He was sniffing around, trying to buy some hot artwork to smuggle back to America, where he intended to resell it and make a killing."

"Okay, go on."

"Well, Niles was certainly in a tight spot. He owed a fortune to the kind of people who take an active dislike to deadbeats. He managed to convince his London creditors—actually, the casino and the loanshark operation were merely different departments of the same operation—to give him a little more time. That was when Niles began negotiations with Weiner, Carlson and Boyd."

"Why didn't he just go to his father?" Morgan asked. "Sam has got all the money in the world."

Nicole shrugged. "Pride, I suppose. From what Niles has told me he's disappointed his father on more than one occasion. I suppose he wanted to get himself out of this mess without daddy's help."

"But Weiner and his firm would never have loaned money to Niles without bringing Sam Kingman into it."

"Probably not," Nicole agreed. "But Niles was frightened. He wasn't thinking clearly. Anyway, when he found out from his contact at Weiner's firm that *you* were in negotiations to borrow money for DonSport's expansion, Niles had his brilliant idea. That's when he recontacted me."

"Where do you fit into all this?"

Nicole smiled, gave him a kiss on the cheek and whispered, "I'm a crook, darling. I act as a go-between, bringing together the buyers and sellers of stolen artwork. That's how I came to know Niles in the first place, to help him buy the stolen art he'd intended to smuggle back to America. When he first arrived in London Niles contacted some people, who knew some people in Paris, who knew me . . ."

"I don't fucking believe this," Morgan blurted. "And your career as a journalist?"

"Is a perfect cover. Oh, I take my writing seriously, but as an added benefit being a free lance journalist allows me to move in all kinds of circles without attracting attention. I was in the midst of putting together a lovely deal for Niles, but then he had to go and lose his borrowed money at the craps table. You know, I do believe he is a compulsive gambler."

"I can't believe it," Morgan slowly said. "That day in Paris, when you were telling me about the whole subject of stolen art, you sounded so adamantly contemptuous of those involved . . ."

She grinned with pleasure. "You said it yourself, darling. I am sneaky, yes?" She kissed him again. "You must understand that all along I thought you were playing a game; I thought you were pretending ignorance of the smuggling scheme, so I went along and pretended as well, thinking it would be the best way to assure you of my reliability."

"All right, go on." Morgan said. "You were telling me about Niles' brilliant idea?"

"He already knew quite a bit about the stolen art network, you see, including the mob's problem getting the stolen art across European borders, and especially into America. And of course, he already knew me," Nicole modestly smiled. "Niles recontacted me, and asked me to present the London mob with a deal: they forgive his debts, and he would supply them with a means to smuggle art into America. Not just a few pieces, but a massive inventory."

"Through *my* company," Morgan grumbled. "That's why he was so adamant about his transport people handling the cars until they reached the DonSport dealerships. He claimed it had to do with unions, but that was a crock of shit. My cars were to be nothing but packing cases for his ripped off statues and whatever."

"Yes, darling. Niles put *Viewpoint* in touch with Weiner's employee, knowing that the employee would leak the information, spoiling your deal," Nicole explained. "Then he just sat back and let you stew for a while, knowing that you'd be ripe for a generous deal when he made his offer to you at the Paris Salon."

"He reeled me in like a fish on the line," Morgan said.

"Of course, I just realized that last part now," she added. "Up until tonight I'd been certain that you were involved in the scheme, despite Niles' boasts about tricking you."

"Because I was looking for money to finance an expansion," Morgan nodded, "Is that why you thought I was in on this?"

"Yes, darling." She shrugged. "Niles told me that neither you nor his father were involved, but I didn't believe him, until now."

"Sam Kingman is an honest man," Morgan said. "No way would he knowingly be involved in this kind of thing. And stop calling me darling," he growled. "You used me, just as Niles did."

"We've used each other, *darling,*" Nicole insisted. "We've used each other in bed, and out of it."

"I'm going to the cops, Nicole."

"Of course, you're not," she told him jovially.

Morgan stood up and began putting on his pants. "Watch me. I'm going to blow the whistle on cowboy Niles, and on you."

"Morgan, listen to me," she said, serious now. "The people whom Niles and I are involved with are very dangerous. If we fail, they would kill Niles, and me." She went to him and put her arms around him. "And even if they didn't, at the very least, it would mean prison for me," she murmured and kissed him.

Morgan hesitated. His hand caressed her cheek.

"Nicole, I'm sorry, I really am," he said softly. "I'll help you any way I can. I'll pay for lawyers, and I'll pay for you to be physically protected, if it comes to that, but I've got to go to the police. I won't break the law."

She pulled away from him. "What about your own life?" she demanded harshly.

Morgan zipped up his pants and reached for his shirt. "I've got nothing to do with any of this, why should your gangster buddies blame me?"

"They'll blame you because they'll think that you were partners with Niles, just as I did. They'll think you backed out, and they'll punish you for it."

Morgan realized she was right. They would believe that he'd been in on the whole damned mess from the beginning. "But I'll be out of their reach in America," he said.

"No you won't," she said confidently. "You'll be right here with Niles and me, in either a French or British prison."

"What are you talking about?" But Morgan knew exactly, and it made him sick to his stomach.

"Will it be either an English jail, or a French one?" She mocked him with a sigh. "It is so hard to say in which you will rot; jurisdiction in these matters gets so tangled."

"Dammit, I'm warning you—"

She laughed in his face. "No, darling. I am warning *you*. You must realize that you are snugly framed into this little endeavor of ours. The authorities would never believe your innocence, not with me testifying that you'd been in on it right from the start."

Morgan swallowed hard. "You'd lie about it to protect Niles?"

Her hard expression softened. "Darling, let's forget about Niles for the moment. You must see that *I* have everything at stake in this matter. Please, you must do exactly as I say. Go along with it just this one time. After that, I'll be out of it, and you can do what you wish."

Sure, Morgan thought. Once he'd broken the law they'd have an even firmer grip on his balls; they could blackmail him into cooperating in their smuggling scheme for as long as they wanted; they could even pin the entire thing on him. After all, DonSport, America was *his* business.

There was no way Morgan was going to go along with this, but he couldn't tell that to Nicole. He'd have to string her along, get her off his back for now, and then try and find a way out of this mess.

"Okay," he said dully. "You win. What do you want me to do?"

Nicole's expression was doubtful. "I wonder if I can trust you . . . if you're smart enough to play it the right way—*my way?*"

"I'll do what you want because I have no choice. You said so, yourself."

"All right," she nodded. "Niles didn't want me to say anything about all of this to you, and now I understand why. You must pretend that this conversation never took place. Niles is the key to everything working out for all of us. The stolen art has been coming over from England in bits and pieces for some time, but only Niles and his London sponsors know where it is hidden now and when it is due to be trucked to Le Mans."

"That's why you've been coming on to me, isn't it?" Morgan asked sadly. "You thought I was Nile's partner in this, which meant that I probably knew where that truckload of goods was. All along, that's what you've really been after?"

"That's not the *only* reason, Morgan," Nicole said softly. "I *do* care for you. We're very good together, darling." She sighed, "But, yes; I must admit that I'm very disappointed, and very worried over the fact that you don't know the truck's whereabouts. You see, I'm worried about Niles. His nerves are stretched to the breaking point. You've got to help me hold Niles together, at least until I learn where that truck is. If Niles breaks, or this scheme falls through, we may

233

escape the law, but if we lose the artwork to the authorities, we'll never escape the mob." She smiled. "Just remember, darling: I'll see to it that anything bad that happens to me will also happen to you." Before she could continue, there was a knock at the door. "Are you expecting someone?" she asked.

"I don't know what to expect anymore," he said sourly. "You're naked," he reminded her. "My robe's hanging in the bathroom." As she went into the bath, he moved to the door and opened it.

"Hello, love of my life!" Sonny, bright eyed and apple cheeked, threw her arms around him, backing him into the room. "Ooh, I like a man without a shirt! He's got less to take off before bed! I would have been here earlier, Morgan, honest I would have, but on the way over I got waylaid by Fabi, and I had to buy him a drink, and guess what? He let me drive the Gatto on the test circuit! It was just fabulous—"

She stopped dead. Her eyes widened, and she went pale as Nicole, barely concealed beneath a bath towel, stepped out of Morgan's bathroom.

"Who is it, darling?" Nicole called out. "Room service with the champagne? Oh! My . . ." Morgan watched helplessly as Nicole pretended surprise and embarrassment, as she smiled mockingly at Sonny, "How are you, dear child?"

"You bastard," Sonny whispered to Morgan. He watched the tears well in her eyes. "You bastard."

Morgan tried to stop her but she tore herself free of his grasp and bolted from the room. Morgan started after her.

"Don't!" Nicole commanded, and something in her voice stopped him in his tracks. "Stay right here," she declared. "We have things to talk about."

He whirled around to confront her. "That business with Sonny wasn't necessary."

"Time for little girls to grow up," Nicole coldly replied. "Now shut that door, and then listen very carefully."

17

SONNY STUMBLED BLINDLY out of the hotel. She brutally repressed her tears, managing to maintain her poise while she waited for the valet to fetch her car. When she was finally settled behind the wheel of the white DeManto coupe, she drove around the corner, out of sight of the hotel, and immediately pulled over.

She sat with the engine idling, in the dark except for the dashboard's glow, and she let herself go. She rested her forehead against the steering wheel and cried and cried, letting out all of her rage and disappointed grief in huge, wracking sobs.

Her chances with Morgan had been slim right from the beginning, she told herself. She could either be grateful or angry about their one night together, but that one night was all there was ever going to be, and she had to face that fact. She couldn't compete with women like Nicole, the sexy, polished, accomplished women of the world who hunted men like Don Morgan.

She thought about going back to her room, but she couldn't face the idea of staring at those four walls. There were plenty of cafes, but they'd all be swarming with reporters. She checked her face in the rearview mirror: her eyes were red and her face was tear streaked; she certainly didn't *look* prepared to face anyone; she knew she didn't *feel* prepared.

The DeManto's gas gauge read three quarters full. She decided to go for a drive. Being in control of a sleek, powerful car always made her feel better, more in control of her life.

Sonny put the DeManto coupe into gear and pulled away from the curb. She drove out of the town on N139, reaching and traveling the first leg of the race circuit, but she bypassed the Mulsanne hairpin bend to continue towards Tours. She was getting out of town. The last thing she wanted was to hang around Le Mans, or anyplace that reminded her of Morgan.

She drove for about fifty kilometers, reveling in the feel of the car and her mastery over it. She was going to learn how to handle her life the way she could handle a set of wheels; she was going to go back home and give Arthur Neal another chance, and if he wasn't the right guy for her, she'd find someone else, but she would *find somebody*, because she wouldn't crawl for *any* man.

She drove hard and fast. Whenever she felt the tears coming on again she'd press down a little harder on the gas pedal, to outrun them. She challenged herself on the dark, unfamiliar, winding road through the Bercé Forest, and then she pushed on, to the Braye River, finally slowing and turning around when she'd reached the sleepy little town of Château-du-loir.

She started back.

It was almost one in the morning. The road was deserted. She was physically and mentally exhausted by the demands of her fast, night sprint, but at least she had also managed to numb her emotions. She knew that wouldn't last. The pain of her broken heart would return to stay with her for a long time to come.

This time around she took it slow through the forest. She had suddenly become so sleepy that her eyes were playing tricks on her. She kept thinking that the heavy woods on either side of the road were harboring animals—deer or whatever—about to leap out in front of her car. One thing was for sure: Sonny wouldn't want to suffer a breakdown around here at this time of night. Talk about deserted . . . she seemed to be all alone in the world.

For that reason it came as a relief when a pair of headlights loomed in her rearview mirror, and began steadily closing. The idea of someone else traveling this road gave her a sense of comradery. Anyway, she was almost out of the woods, literally, if not emotionally; another twenty kilometers and she'd be back in Le Mans and could go to bed.

"What the—" Sonny winced, squinting in the sudden blaze of light as the car behind her threw on its high beams and suddenly zoomed up, to just kiss the DeManto's rear bumper.

Sonny clicked on her right turn signal, and took her foot off the gas. She angled over towards the shoulder. If this jerk was so anxious to pass, she was even more anxious to let him.

The big car—Sonny couldn't be sure, but she thought it was a Mercedes 500S series—glided up parallel, then edged its nose a little past the DeManto, and began to angle in towards Sonny. Whoever was in that car was trying to "bulldog" her, force her to reduce her speed until they had her stopped—and trapped.

Sonny didn't know what this was all about, but she had no intention of letting anyone get to her in this dark and deserted place. If their car was a Mercedes 500, they'd have about the top speed of her DeManto, and a hell of a lot more heft in a bumper-car encounter, but nowhere near her nimble little coupé's maneuverability in a flat-out chase. She decided to make a run for it. Maybe she'd get lucky, and they'd cross the path of some cop making his sleepy-eyed night rounds.

She waited for the road to somewhat straighten out, and then lightly touched the DeManto's brakes. The intercepting car shot past, its own brake lights glowing cherry red. Now the car was clearly illuminated in Sonny's headlights, and she saw that she'd been right; it was a silver Mercedes 560SEL.

But now that she was momentarily clear of her pursuers and out of danger of a collision, it was time to say good-bye.

Sonny stood on the brakes, turning the steering wheel hard to the left, at the same time jamming the DeManto into reverse. As the coupé's rear end whipped around into the opposite lane, its engine, transmission, and tires all screeching in a chorus of pain, she jabbed the stick into first and peeled out. Her stomach felt like it was braided around her spine, and she'd taken about a hundred thousand miles off the life of the car, but the split second "J-turn" now had her traveling in the opposite direction from the Mercedes. She was no longer heading back toward Le Mans, but at least she was free!

She was pumped up now. There was about a gallon of adrenalin coursing through her system. She was wide awake, alert, and at her driving peak. No way those assholes in their German tank were going to catch Sonny Thomas; not when she was in a DeManto, and not on this road—

The high beams coming out of nowhere several hundred feet ahead of her filled Sonny's windshield with dazzling motes of light and almost sent her hurtling into the trees. She slowed down as she watched another fucking Mercedes, this one light blue, come to a stop angled across both lanes, effectively blocking the road. She tried to play chicken with this second car, making it seem like she was going to slam into them, but when it looked like they weren't going to fall for it, she braked hard and performed another J-turn back toward Le Mans, in time to see the first Mercedes duplicate the other car's maneuver: they had her boxed in.

Sonny stomped on the gas pedal, intending to steer around the first car, driving on the shoulder and sideswiping trees if she had to. As she peeled out, the coupé's rear end fishtailing under the sudden acceleration, Sonny suddenly felt her steering go heavy, and heard that dismal *whoppity-whoppity* sound. More disgusted than frightened, she stopped the car. She'd blown both rear tires.

Four men got out of the Mercedes in front of her. Sonny, watching them approach in the glare of her headlights, saw that they were dressed in suits and ties. She glanced in the rearview mirror and saw three more men approaching, starkly silhouetted against the sidespill of the rear Mercedes' lights. She listened to the ill-tempered mutterings of her idling, disabled car, and thought about making a run for it on foot, but she didn't think much of her chances of eluding seven men in these dark and unfamiliar woods.

One of the men coming up from the rear approached her side of the crippled DeManto and tapped at the driver's window with what Sonny at first took to be an extraordinarily long-barreled target pistol. Then she rolled down her window realizing that she'd seen enough spy movies to recognize a silenced automatic pistol when she saw one.

Like the others, this man was impeccably dressed. He was totally bald. Sonny could see the stubble on the sides of his head from where he'd shaved away the little hair he'd had left. He had dark, bushy eyebrows and a matching moustache. He pointed his futuristic looking gun in no particular direction and said in heavily French accented English, *"Mademoiselle,* please realize that I could shoot you as easily as I shot your tires."

"No argument, there," Sonny wisecracked with bravado she certainly didn't feel. The guy's manner was so quiet and polite; it spooked her more than if he'd come on tough and threatening. He didn't seem at all involved or concerned with what he was doing; as if running people off the road and shooting out their tires with a silenced automatic was all in a day's work. "Tell me," Sonny asked brightly, "to what do I owe the pleasure of this hijacking?"

"Actually, this is a kidnapping, *mademoiselle*." He opened Sonny's door. "Get out of your car and come with us, if you please."

As Sonny reached to shut off the DeManto's engine, the man said, "Please leave the keys in the ignition. We will dispose of your car."

"Nice of you." Sonny got out of the car. Her heart was pounding and her legs felt rubbery weak. She couldn't help gasping and flinching as two of the men closed in, each taking a firm hold of one of her arms. They marched her towards the silver Mercedes, the man with the gun taking the lead, another man in the rear. They put her in the backseat, still bracketed by the two men. The man with the pistol got in on the front passenger's side. As the driver put the Mercedes in gear and headed toward Le Mans, the man with the gun twisted around in his seat and said, "The man next to you is about to inject you with a sedative, *mademoiselle*."

"No!" she cried out. She had been moving through this experience as if it were a dream, but she was truly panicked now, ready to fight for her life. "I don't want it! No!" She struggled, but it was useless. The man with the gun held a pencil flashlight on her as the two men on either side of her firmly immobilized her arm and pushed up her sleeve.

"Do not be afraid. It will only make you sleep," the man with the gun said in his chatty manner. He didn't smile, or gloat; he didn't frown. "It is for your own good, *mademoiselle*. And if I may put it frankly, you have no choice in the matter."

She smelled rubbing alcohol, and watched them swab cotton against her skin, then felt a pinprick as the hypo slid into her vein.

Light blue liquid left the syringe and went into her arm. She had time to think that it looked like Tidy Bowl treated toilet water; they were shooting her up with *fucking Tidy Bowl;* and then she didn't seem to be thinking of anything at all.

18

MORGAN BEGAN CALLING Sonny's hotel room as soon as Nicole had left him. He called every fifteen minutes, and as time ticked away, and it got to be one, then two in the morning, he considered calling the police. He would have, had the missing person been anyone but Sonny Thomas. Instead he called down to the garage and found out that her car was gone.

He knew her habits pretty well; she was out driving to blow off steam. He'd give her a little longer before making things even more complicated by calling the cops. Besides, Nicole might find out about his calling the authorities and misconstrue his actions. He didn't know what he was going to do to extricate himself from the mess he'd gotten himself into, but before he could deal with it he had to straighten things out with Sonny.

And while he was waiting for her, Morgan, yawning, decided to stretch out for a little while on the bed. He didn't think that he'd be able to sleep, but he did. His life was so incredibly fucked up that there was nothing, or too much, for him to think about. He drifted right off.

The ringing phone jolted him out of his doze. He stabbed at the receiver, at the same time looking at his watch: three thirty. "Sonny?" he mumbled, still half asleep. "You okay?"

"It's me."

"Nicole?"

"Morgan, listen to me very carefully. After I left you, I thought about our conversation, and I decided that I wasn't totally convinced that you would do as I'd said. I decided to take out a little insurance on the matter. "I've got Sonny."

"You *kidnapped* her?" Morgan blurted, shocked, and now very wide awake. "You bitch! If she's hurt, I'll hurt *you.*"

"She has not been hurt," Nicole impatiently replied.

"And I'll go to the cops! You tell whoever is holding her that I don't care if I go to prison along with the bunch of you—"

"Shut up!" Nicole snapped. "Save your idle threats. I told you, she has not been hurt, and she will not be, as long as you cooperate. But, I warn you, the people who have her are professionals. Do you understand? This is not a game to them. They kill people as a matter of course. They would find your blustering even more laughable than I do. Sonny is being well cared for now, but all that could change in an instant if you make trouble."

Morgan realized that Nicole was right. For Sonny's sake, he had to play along. "What do I have to do?" Morgan asked, forcing meekness into his tone.

"That's better," Nicole said smugly. "Do just what I told you. Act perfectly normal with Niles Kingman, and stay out of my hair."

"When will Sonny be released?"

"I don't know," Nicole replied. "Honestly, I don't. That truckload of artwork may arrive tomorrow, or it may arrive the day of the race. Niles must remain calm until it gets here. Once I've got it, he becomes rather less important to the operation. At that point Sonny will be released, unharmed." Her voice became harsh. "Now all you have to do is behave yourself. Play this smart. Do not even think of going to the police. It would mean Sonny's death, and I'd still see to it that I took you along to prison." She laughed, "Perhaps they'd allow us to share a cell, darling," and hung up.

Morgan put down the receiver and collapsed back onto the bed. He bleakly stared up at the ceiling. He was hopelessly outclassed. Like Nicole had said, he was up against professionals.

He'd lost.

There was no way that he was going to come out of this unscathed, but he didn't matter. Not even to himself, he realized. The only person he cared about was Sonny. He would cooperate with Niles, and Nicole, and the rest of these crooks; he'd become a crook himself, helping them to smuggle their goods into America in his cars. He'd do anything he had to do, as long as Sonny was safe.

Just please, let that goddamned truck come tomorrow, and then Sonny would be out of it.

Morgan dozed fitfully through what was left of the night. By morning he was showered, shaved, and dressed, and not the least bit sleepy—just sick to his stomach over what the coming day might bring.

At nine he called down for his car and drove over to the Le Mans circuit for his first appointment of the day. All that morning and for most of the afternoon he felt like a zombie going through the motions, not really there through the organizational conferences and media interviews. *When the fuck was that truck going to come?* he obsessed. *When would Sonny be released?*

Nicole, smiling and efficient and deceitful, was around for the first part of the day, and then, thankfully, she disappeared. Morgan could no longer endure the sight of her. Niles Kingman stuck around. His Stetson was a beacon Morgan avoided as much as possible.

It was around five in the afternoon, and Morgan was taking advantage of a break in his schedule, having coffee at the cafe by the circuit stands. He was sitting at an outside table in the dying sunshine, brooding about a thousand things, all of which boiled down to the fact that once again, despite his best efforts, his life and the lives of those he touched were falling to pieces, right here at Le Mans. It was as if this place held some awful curse for him. He'd caused the death of Lee Thomas here. Now he was in danger of killing Lee's daughter. Hell, the only thing different about the situation this time around was that he wasn't drinking. Shit, he might as *well* be . . .

He knocked back his espresso, threw some francs down on the table, and left the cafe. All he could think about was Sonny.

He felt strong and whole when he was with her.

Just let her survive, and he would tell her that, Morgan vowed.

He walked past the paddock's front gates. It gave him some satisfaction to see that the enclosed area was crowded with spectators gawking at the participating cars that were on display. By tradition, the paddock area was open to the public before a race to let them have a chance to get a close-up look at the machinery. Ironically, it looked as if the race and the DonSport, America kickoff was going to be a huge success, for everyone but Don Morgan and Sonny Thomas.

He kept on walking to where he'd parked his car by the stands. He was meeting his next appointment at the Cafe du Tertre Rouge, a stone cottage in the wooded grove by the Tertre Rouge bend of the racing circuit—

"*Monsieur* Morgan!"

Morgan turned around as three unfamiliar looking men in business suits and ties walked briskly towards him.

"*Monsieur*, you will come with us, please," said the guy in the lead, who was bald with bushy eyebrows and a moustache.

"Come with you where?" Morgan stared at him. "What's going on?"

"You will come with us, right now." Baldy said pleasantly, but forcefully.

These are Nicole's people, Morgan realized. He was being kidnapped. He felt slow and stupid; he didn't know what to do. He wanted to run, but while he'd been standing around with his jaw hanging, the three had formed a loose circle around him, fencing him in. He struggled to shake off the shock and think clearly. He *had* to think clearly.

"Monsieur, cooperate, if you please," Baldy said reasonably. His face was expressionless as he opened up his suit jacket to show Morgan the butt of a pistol in a shoulder holster. "Cause no commotion, and walk away with us. Right now."

Morgan looked around. There were people everywhere, but it was getting dark. At any instant these guys could stick a knife into him and no one would be the wiser. But he couldn't call out for help. These guys still had Sonny. Anyway, an incident between himself and a trio of goons would certainly be enough to spook Niles.

But if *he* couldn't make a scene, neither could these guys . . . Morgan smiled. "Guess what, Mister Clean? I'm not going anywhere with you assholes." He turned around, shouldered his way through the two guys blocking him and began to stride away. He wasn't sure where he was going, but then he spotted Niles Kingman's cowboy hat. Niles was talking with some guy just inside the paddock's front gate. Morgan made a beeline that way.

"Monsieur, stop now! Please, I warn you—" Baldy urgently whispered as he followed right on Morgan's heels.

"Fuck you, pal," Morgan growled. "In case you don't know, that's everybody's favorite bundle of raw nerves, Niles Kingman, straight ahead. You want to shoot me, go right ahead. You want to try and take me by force, that's fine. But before you do anything, maybe you'd better check with Nicole, because old Niles might just decide to screw-up a certain special delivery if you spook him."

Morgan felt an ironlike grip clamping his arm. Baldy hissed, "You fool, stop—"

Morgan pulled free and dashed the remaining few

paces to the gate. "Niles, a word with you, buddy!" Morgan called out heartily, not looking back, expecting a bullet, a shiv, a karate chop—not knowing what to expect.

"Jeez, Morgan," Kingman scowled. "I'm in the middle of somethin' here with this guy from *Forbes*. Can't it wait?"

"Not really," Morgan said, glancing over his shoulder. The trio of goons were standing about fifty feet away, staring at him. "I'd like to speak with you, alone."

"What's up?" Niles demanded, stepping away from the reporter. "That was an important interview . . ." his voice trailed off as he looked past Morgan, to stare uneasily at the goons, who abruptly walked away.

"Who are those guys?" Niles asked, as behind him the paddock's floodlights flickered on to augment the setting sun's purplish light.

Kingman sounded shaky, Morgan thought. He really *was* a nervous wreck. Morgan remembered Nicole's warning about upsetting the man and realized that Sonny's life depended on how fast and convincingly Morgan could spin some lies. "Those guys work for one of the auto manufacturers who refused to take part in our race."

"They work for a carmaker?" Niles, repeated, sounding bewildered.

"Sure, you see, they were trying to talk me into canceling this whole event."

Niles tightly gripped Morgan's sleeve. "You can't do that. We've got a deal. I need this race to—"

"Hey, take it easy," Morgan laughed. "Nobody's canceling anything. They're just a couple of disgruntled auto execs, Niles. Don't sweat it. The only reason I came over to talk to you was to get clear of them."

Morgan watched Kingman struggle to calm down. "Okay . . ." He took a deep breath. "No problem." He glanced at his watch. "Morgan, I've got to get back to that reporter."

"Yeah, good idea, Niles," Morgan soothed. "The more publicity the better."

"I'll see you later." Kingman cast one final, worried glance at the three men, who'd returned to loiter nearby. "You take care of yourself, Morgan."

"Yeah, okay." Morgan watched the Three Stooges start to close in on him again as soon as he was alone. He began to walk away from the paddock, towards the pit garages near the stands, figuring that at least the garages were well-lit, and crowded, and not open to the public. He could get inside, but his three friends on his tail couldn't.

Nicole had sent these goons, Morgan knew. She'd had Sonny kidnapped, and now she was trying to nab him. It made sense. She was the career crook; she was the one willing to cut and run with the stolen goods should Niles' smuggling plan fall through.

And if she were making a move against Morgan, it could only mean that he was no longer necessary. It could only mean that she *had* that truckload of art.

Shit, it really *did* make sense. Nicole was like the proverbial rat deserting the sinking ship. Now that she knew that Morgan was an unwitting and unwilling participant in Nile's scheme, she knew that the complicated smuggling plan would never hold together. She'd probably decided to grab the artwork—she obviously had the manpower to do it—as soon as she'd discovered the truth about Morgan. She intended to leave Niles Kingman empty handed, leave him to try to explain things to the London faction represented by those British toughs masquerading as Kingman and Son transport workers.

The only reason Nicole had kidnapped Sonny was to keep him from either calling the cops or tipping off Niles, Morgan now realized. As he entered the safety of the bustling, DeManto garage, leaving his tail waiting for him outside, he realized one other thing: that he was out of this smuggling mess. Just like that he was out of it. Entirely.

Niles would be taken care of by a very angry, stung, London mob. Nicole, the proud owner of a fortune in stolen art, certainly wasn't about to implicate Morgan to the police. The worst that was going to happen was that Sam Kingman was going to be too busy mourning the sudden untimely death or disappearance of his prodigal son to want to continue with the expansion deal.

But Nicole's goons still had Sonny, Morgan knew. And they were still after him. Evidently Nicole had decided it would be best not to leave any loose ends lying around . . .

Morgan knew that Sonny was still alive. He desperately wanted to believe it, but it also made sense. Right now, Nicole and her band of goons were smugglers. They would not want to risk a murder charge unless they were absolutely positive that they were going to get away clean. That was why they were trying to nab *him.* They would not harm Sonny while there was still a chance that he might go to the police and blow the entire thing wide open. But once they had him, both he and Sonny could be killed, and there would be no one around to point an accusing finger at free lance journalist Nicole Houel, except for Niles, and he couldn't point at her from the grave, or, assuming the unlikely possibility that the London mob was merciful and spared him, without also pointing at himself.

That meant the goons would either grab or simply out-and-out murder him at their first opportunity, but Morgan knew that he couldn't go to the police. If he did, his own safety would be assured, but Nicole and her people might panic and kill Sonny—

Unless Morgan had a hostage of his own, someone who could directly link Nicole to Sonny's disappearance and cause Nicole to think twice before she did anything foolish. Niles could implicate Nicole in the smuggling scheme, but he was a dead end, in more ways than one, as far as Sonny's kidnapping was concerned. About the kidnapping, he knew even less than Morgan.

No, if he wanted to save Sonny, he was going to have to get hold of someone who was likely to be directly involved in the kidnapping, someone who could pin it directly on Nicole.

Like, say, Baldy, for instance . . .

Morgan went back to the garage entrance and peeked out. Baldy and one of his back-up were standing across the way, waiting for him to leave.

Baldy even waved at him. *Cocky sonofabitch,* Morgan thought, and went back inside.

Fabiano Manfredi, in a white lab coat, clipboard in hand, was chatting with some of his mechanics, beside a Gatto. The back-up Gatto was on display to the public at the paddock.

"Fabi, I need this car," Morgan said.

"Donaldo, it is not possible," Manfredi complained. "This car is for the race, tomorrow."

"Look, I haven't got time to argue."

"What if something happens to it?"

"Something *is* going to happen to it," Morgan replied. "But don't worry. You've got the other one."

"Donaldo, the other one is not like this one," Manfredi slyly winked, patting the sleek, blood-red convertible's hood.

Morgan stared at him. "Fabi, did you have your boys modify this car?"

"Just a little bit, Donaldo," Manfredi cajoled, twirling the ends of his handlebar moustache like a silent movie villain. "We did some engine work, played with the turbo, and replaced the suspension, sway bars, and brakes." He offered Morgan his typically Italian shrug. "We must win this race, my friend. For the *Professore,* yes?"

"No!" Morgan adamantly replied. "The rules call for you to enter a street legal, showroom version of this car into the competition, and that's what you're going to do, Fabi. I've had enough cheating this one night to last me my entire life. You'll enter the other unmodified Gatto, and I'll check it myself before the race, and that's final."

"*Si*. Donaldo," Manfredi sighed. "If you insist."

"I insist. Now, give me the keys to this one."

Manfredi shook his head. "I cannot risk this car, my friend. *Especially not* when it is modified the way it is. The *Professore* would never forgive me. It is worth—"

"Two hundred thousand, right?" Morgan demanded impatiently. He pulled a checkbook out of his sport jacket's breast pocket. "You got a pen, Fabi?"

Manfredi wordlessly nodded, pulling a Bic stickpen out of the top of his clipboard.

"Two hundred grand, you said," Morgan muttered, beginning to write.

"Actually, no, I did *not* say," Manfredi said apologetically. "When one takes into account the modifications we made, and the potential damage to the DeManto reputation should our tinkering come to light with the public, I would say that the price of *this* car is more like *three* hundred thousand. *Si*, Donaldo?"

Morgan scowled at him. "I'd haggle for mudflaps and carpet mats, but I'm a little pressed for time." He wrote the check, tore it out of the register, and stuffed it into the breast pocket of Manfredi's lab coat. "There, now you can truthfully claim that this car was never meant to be raced tomorrow, because it's my personal vehicle. Now gas up this fucker, and give me the keys!"

Manfredi, shrugging, rattled off the orders in Italian to his personnel. "Where are you going in such a hurry?"

Morgan gave him a humorless grin. "Sonny's waiting."

He tooled the Gatto slowly out of the garage, wanting to give Baldy and his one remaining sidekick the chance to see him and get wheels of their own. It didn't take long. Morgan was slowly cruising away as a silver Mercedes 560SEL pulled up, and Baldy and his buddy hopped in.

Morgan drove carefully through the crowds, past the paddock and the entrance to the Bugatti Circuit, under the Dunlop Bridge, to the Le Tetre Rouge Bend. He thought briefly about his stood-up appointment at the nearby cafe as he waited at the start of the Mulsanne Straight, to let the Mercedes pull in close. He watched the headlights grow in the rearview mirror; watched until he could actually see Baldy, who was seated in the Mercedes' front passenger's side.

Then Morgan floored the Gatto. The V-12's throaty roar sang in counterpoint to the turbo wail as he took the four wheel drive car smoothly through the gears, hurtling down the straightaway. The Mercedes was no slouch in its own right, but it had no chance against the Gatto. Morgan watched in his rearview mirror as its headlights shrank down to twin fireflies. Morgan clicked on his own high beams: the broken white line down the road's center looked continuous, and the trees along either side were a solid green blur. Within less than fifteen seconds the Gatto's speedometer read 220 kph; about 140 miles per hour. Morgan concentrated on his driving, adroitly weaving through the fortunately sparse traffic on this public stretch of road.

As he reached the end of the straight he slowed down, to give the Mercedes a chance to see him take the Mulsanne Bend. The Gatto's modified brakes slowed the car a lot more quickly, and its stiffened, heavy duty suspension let Morgan feel every ant corpse on the macadam, but otherwise the car was pretty much the vehicle he'd driven from Paris.

He glimpsed the Mercedes darting through the traffic after him. He let it get a good look at his flashing brake lights, and then began to accelerate, but this time not full out. He wanted to tantalize those bastards chasing him. Get them a little frustrated, nice and hot, before he stuck it in. He let them get teasingly close near the Indianapolis Bend of the Le Mans circuit, and then pulled away. At the Arnage bend, he swerved off the Le Mans circuit, and began to fly down the tree lined D139, again, watching out for traffic. His turnoff would be coming up in a few seconds, so he slowed down, to make sure that the Mercedes would see him take it. When the turnoff came, Morgan braked, and swung the Gatto into a hard, right turn, double-clutch downshifting to smoothly make the transition from pavement onto this bumpy dirt road. He knew where he was going. Years ago, during happier times, he had taken girls up along this deserted, heavily wooded, stretch of country lane. He knew that a normal car could handle the ruts and jolts—just not as well and as quickly, as the full time, four wheel drive Gatto.

He could see the Mercedes headlights behind him. He purposely lost the pursuit car at a bend in the road, and then accelerated to the left hand turnaround spot fenced in by a stone wall, that had been his destination all along. Morgan nosed the Gatto into it, hitting the parking brake to lock just the front wheels, while twisting the steering wheel. The stone wall loomed and gravel flew, but Morgan accomplished the maneuver with just inches to spare. He'd executed a perfect 180-degree "bootlegger's turn," so that the Gatto was now facing out, towards the road. Morgan killed the lights, tightened his seatbelt, and waited.

He saw the Mercedes' stabbing high beams, before he saw the car. He rolled down the window and listened. As he'd hoped, it sounded like it was rattling along at about 35 mph, far too fast for a heavy, rear wheel drive car on such an awful road; even a superb car like the Mercedes 560SEL. He could hear it bouncing and bucking on its suspension; it sounded as if it was off balance, at the limits of its rolling traction.

Morgan clicked on his high beams, threw the Gatto into first and stomped it, all in the instant before the Mercedes' nose came into view. He was pushed back into his seat by the G-force as the powerful four wheel drive car bit into the dirt and literally pounced out of its hiding place, rocketing across the road. Morgan steered to "T-bone" the Mercedes, striking the car broadside just behind the front left fender, plowing into it with a deafening crash.

Morgan, tightly belted into the Gatto's contoured bucket seat, was prepared for the impact; the Mercedes' passengers were not. The driver threw up his hands, letting go of the steering wheel. There was the screech of sheet metal rending, and the grinding noise of tires spinning as the Gatto struggled to move the heavier vehicle off course. As Morgan had hoped, his speed, and the fact that the big Mercedes was off balance, allowed him to plow it off the road, head-on into a tree.

As the Mercedes front end telescoped, stopping all further movement, the Gatto's engine stalled, and Morgan felt himself lurch forward against his shoulder harness. He settled back into the bucket seat scared and oddly giddy, but physically unharmed.

Things got quiet very quickly. With both cars dead, there was only the clicking of hot metal, and the sigh of steam escaping from the crumpled engine compartments. Morgan jumped out of the Gatto, its bashed-in nose mashed flat against the sagging driver's door of the other car, and ran around to the passenger's side of the Mercedes. As he jerked open the door, the Mercedes overhead lamp went on, and Baldy spilled out onto the ground. Morgan quickly glanced inside; both the driver, floating face down in the blossomed air bag, and the backseat passenger, who was lying sprawled on the carpeted floor, seemed to be out cold. Baldy, looking dazed, was slowly trying to crawl away. Morgan knelt down and flipped him over onto his back. The man had a bad gash across his cheek; blood was spilling down along the side of his nose, into his mouth. He tried to grab at Morgan, who slapped his hands away, and then reached inside his suit jacket to snatch away his gun.

There were moans coming from inside the Mercedes as Morgan stared at the big, matte black automatic with its black plastic grips. He knew a little about guns from his Army stint, but that had been rifles, and a hell of a long time ago. The guy in the backseat was sitting up as Morgan thumbed what he thought was the safety catch, revealing a red dot. Okay, Morgan thought. Next question: single action or double action? He pointed the gun at a tree and pulled the trigger. The weapon bucked in his hand; he heard the crack, and by the Mercedes' interior light, saw the ejected brass shell casing go spinning away into the darkness.

"Okay!" Morgan yelled ferociously. He hadn't felt this wired in years. He pressed the gun against the side of Baldy's head and yelled at the guy in the backseat, "You there! Stay inside that car!" Actually, the guy had seemed in no great hurry to come out since Morgan had fired that shot.

Morgan shifted his attention to Baldy. "You kidnapped Sonny, didn't you?" Baldy looked about to pass out. Morgan slapped him awake with his free hand. "Pay attention!"

Morgan could hear the two-note song of sirens approaching. Somebody must have heard the crash, and called the authorities. All right; he'd accomplished what he'd set out to do. He'd captured three of Nicole's people. He only hoped that this was enough of Nicole's gang to make her think twice before turning a smuggling charge into murder by harming Sonny.

"Just lie still. I'm turning you over to the police," Morgan told Baldy.

Baldy laughed. His smile was blood stained. "We *are* the police."

19

MORGAN PUT THE gun down and stood with his hands in plain view. The dirt road was filling up with Renaults, all with revolving blue lights on their roofs, a pair of ambulances, and an unmarked windowless van. Morgan had thought that Baldy was delirious, or trying to pull a bluff, but when the *gendarmes* carried away the three men like fallen heroes, and snapped the cuffs on *him*, he began to think that maybe he'd made a little mistake.

They put him in the back of the windowless van and drove him somewhere: it turned out to be back to Le Mans, where they unloaded him at the backdoor of the police station. They ignored his pleas concerning Sonny's kidnapping, and his own demands to be allowed to call someone, and put him into a windowless holding room with pale green walls, a bench, a toilet, and nothing else.

He watched the hour hand creep around his Rolex. He thought about how he had no idea what was going on, but whatever it was, it was a good bet that it wasn't what he'd thought. They finally came back for him at about nine thirty. He'd been locked up over three hours, and he was ripping. The fact that the two uniformed cops who marched him out of the room were still ignoring his questions did not help to calm him.

The two cops took him down a flight of steps, and along a fluorescent-lit basement corridor. Morgan stopped being angry and began to get scared. If what Baldy had said about being a cop was true, who knew what these guys were planning?

They took him into what looked like the station's lunchroom: more fluorescent light fixtures, high, windowless, cinder-block walls, a row of vending machines, and lots of long, folding tables surrounded by those candy-colored, plastic stackable chairs. Niles Kingman, wearing handcuffs and looking pale, was seated at one of the tables, under the watchful eyes of a couple of uniformed cops. At a nearby table, an obviously distraught Sam Kingman sat conferring with a bunch of serious looking guys in suits.

Over on the far side of the room, half a dozen plainclothes cops, some of them with their suit jackets off to reveal their shoulder holsters, were pushing pencils at a table littered with folders and glossy photographs. The cops were smiling and joking among themselves in French. Right there with them, chatting and shuffling papers just like one of the boys, was Nicole Houel.

She moved away from the table to meet Morgan as the cops brought him over. "Before you say anything," she began, "Know that Sonny is safe. She always has been."

Morgan looked at the cops clustered around the table. "They look like they're enjoying their work. I guess you got your truckload of stolen art?"

"It was a magnificent bust, darling. We pulled our raid an hour ago. I'm so sorry we had to keep you locked up, but we couldn't chance you going to the press, and there was nobody to explain things to you." She smiled. "Your valiant attempt to counter Sonny's kidnapping did leave us a little shorthanded at a crucial time." She turned to the pair of cops who had escorted him downstairs. Morgan listened to her excuse them in French.

The policemen nodded deferentially and went away. "So, you're a cop, huh?" Morgan asked bleakly.

"Interpol agent," Nicole replied. She gestured towards a silver-haired man in his sixties in a dark blue suit, chewing on a curved stem, black briar pipe as he bent over the table, studying the photographs. "That's my superior, Inspector Danner."

Danner looked up, nodded once, and went back to his pictures.

"Those three guys in the Mercedes?"

"Interpol agents," Nicole wryly nodded.

"So, I crashed a three hundred thousand dollar car into a seventy thousand dollar car full of police officers."

"I'm sorry about the damage to your beautiful car. The policemen were not seriously injured," Nicole said. "Your actions were foolhardy, but somewhat understandable under the circumstances—"

"Somewhat understandable!" Morgan shouted. Everybody glanced at him, but Morgan didn't care; he figured he was entitled to lose his cool. "You, and Interpol, ought to be thankful those guys are okay, because if they weren't, it would have been your fault, not mine!"

Inspector Danner looked disapprovingly at Morgan and went back to his work.

"Well, what am I charged with?" Morgan asked as he pulled out a chair and sat down.

"Nothing!" Nicole said adamantly. "This entire operation is off the record. You were never brought here, and Interpol was never here."

"Right." Morgan massaged his temples with his fingertips. "What's going to happen is that any second now I'm going to wake up and I'm going to be back in Kansas."

"Morgan, please let me explain," Nicole began.

"I can't wait to hear you explain, Mata Hari, but first tell me where Sonny is?"

"As I said, she's safe and sound," Nicole replied, sounding a little miffed.

"Wonderful, now you're a jealous Interpol agent.

257

Stop playing games with me!" Morgan jumped to his feet. "I want answers, now!"

One of the plainclothes cops took a step in their direction. Nicole shook her head, and the cop went back to his paperwork after casting Morgan a baleful glare.

"Sonny is only a kilometer or so from here," Nicole quickly explained. "She is staying in the home of the police surgeon here in Le Mans. We put her there merely to keep her out of sight. And since we'd administered the sedative we thought—"

"*What* sedative?" Morgan demanded. He shook his head. "This is nuts. I want to see Sonny right now!"

"All in good time."

"And then I'm going to call my lawyers in the States and start suing the ass off of Interpol, and the Le Mans police department, and this doctor buddy of yours who you claim shot her up with dope, and anyone else I can think of."

"Hear me out," Nicole said. "After that, you'll be free to go see Sonny, and you can sue anyone you want to sue, yes?"

"*Yes,*" Morgan mimicked. "I'll listen, but first of all, level with me. Just *who* and *what* are you, Nicole?" He frowned. "*If* that's your name?"

"My name really is Nicole Houel," she laughed, "And I really am a journalist, and involved in the stolen art scene, but that's my cover as an Interpol agent. The story I told you last night, and my role in all of it, is true, except for the fact that I'm an undercover law enforcement officer. It all happened just as I told you. I was put in touch with Niles because of his interest in buying some stolen art to take back to America, but then that deal fell through when he'd gambled away the money he'd borrowed."

"Okay, so far," Morgan nodded.

"Niles did really come to me asking if I'd convince the London mob to let him repay his debts by setting up

258

his smuggling scheme using DonSport. Interpol instructed me to help Niles achieve his goal. We knew that we had to play along. Here was the London mob about to give us the opportunity to regain virtually their entire inventory of stolen art. As I told you, up until last night I was certain that you and Niles' father were involved. After I'd tipped my hand to you, and found out I was wrong, I realized that I'd unwittingly put Interpol's entire operation in jeopardy." She smiled apologetically. "I had to act tough with you. I couldn't let you upset Niles. We might have lost the shipment of goods."

"Why did you feel you had to grab Sonny?" Morgan demanded.

"I am afraid that was my decision, Mr. Morgan," Inspector Danner interrupted, leaving the table to join them. "Last night Agent Houel reported to me directly after her conversation with you, and her unexpected confrontation with Sonny Thomas, in your hotel room. It was my feeling that one loose cannon—you, sir— rattling around on board ship was enough. Also, as I'm sure you'll agree, having you believe that Miss Thomas was in peril, kept you in line."

"But what's all this about sedating her?" Morgan demanded.

"As long as we were going to feign Miss Thomas' abduction, I thought I should take the opportunity to use the scenario to help strengthen Agent Houel's cover as a criminal," Danner replied, pausing to use a lighter to get his pipe going. "I had her reveal her kidnap plan to those representatives of the London mob who'd come here to keep an eye on their loot."

"Those tough guys pretending to be Kingman transport workers?" Morgan asked.

"Yes," Danner nodded. "Agent Houel told the London faction that she was nabbing Sonny Thomas to keep you in line. The idea was to make her seem ruthless and ready to do anything."

"Actually, it wasn't to have been a staged kidnap at all," Nicole added. "We were merely going to have a police car pick her up—no muss, no fuss." She shrugged. "Things went wrong when one of the London boys suggested that instead of my fooling with Sonny, they would get tough with you. Well, obviously I couldn't let that happen. I reminded them that if you were roughed up, you might not be able to participate in the race. They agreed to leave you out of it, but one of their people insisted on coming along when I had Sonny nabbed."

"Accordingly, the kidnapping had to seem real," Danner said, puffing on his pipe.

"I scrambled to round up some Interpol agents to stage the snatch. I'm afraid that our men had to play a little rough with Sonny for the benefit of our English observer," Nicole apologized. "We had to make it look like a real abduction, right down to injecting her with a mild sedative to keep her quiet and under control."

"That's just fucking great," Morgan glowered.

"But a trained paramedic administered the drug," Nicole quickly added. "She was *never* in any real danger. As soon as we got rid of that English gangster by handing him a story about stashing her in a country house, she went right to the police surgeon's residence."

"But why did you try to kidnap me?" Morgan asked.

"Again, that action was taken upon my orders," Inspector Danner replied. "Nicole thought she had you in hand, but I didn't want to take any chances. By four this afternoon we had the truck pinpointed, but we needed time to set up the raid in a way that wouldn't compromise Agent Houel's cover, or implicate Niles Kingman."

"You were worried about Niles?" Morgan challenged in disbelief.

"We had to protect him," Danner nodded, gesturing with his pipe at the handcuffed man. "You'll understand why in a moment. Getting back to why we decided to nab you . . . Well, we were on the final countdown. It was absolutely crucial that Niles Kingman suspect nothing. Agent Houel felt you would do as you were told, but I believed you were too unpredictable. So I issued orders that you be quietly picked up." The Inspector looked rueful, "That was when we found out just how unpredictable you could be."

"Morgan, why *did* you choose to confront those men," Nicole asked.

Morgan filled them in on his line of reasoning.

"You've got quite an imagination, Mr. Morgan." Inspector Danner grinned when Morgan was done.

"Yeah, you should talk, Sherlock," Morgan grumbled. "This might have been some kind of game for you, but it wasn't exactly fun for me, and it definitely wasn't fun for Sonny. And it easily could have ended in tragedy. At one point I had a loaded gun pressed against a man's head. What if he had made a move, or if I had just overreacted? Who'd have been responsible for that murder?"

"You wouldn't have been charged," Nicole murmured.

"That's not the point," Morgan glared at her. "There's legal responsibility, sure, but then there's—" Both Nicole and Danner were looking at him strangely. "Forget it." Morgan took a deep breath and turned away, shaking his head. "You know, I can forgive everything, but not the way you toyed with Sonny's life. I *am* going to the media with this," Morgan stared at them. "And if I can, I intend to sue—"

"Don, I'm going to ask you to reconsider," Sam Kingman said, coming up to him.

"Why, Sam?" Morgan asked, puzzled.

"They've offered Niles a deal," Sam said, looking embarrassed. "It'll be risky for him, but it's more than he deserves. From what I've just been told by those fellows from Interpol, they managed to use local cops to get what they were after and round up those London thugs. Agent Houel and my son were left out of it."

"That way I can still function undercover," Nicole explained. "It also allows us to offer Niles a deal."

"As of now nobody knows that Niles was arrested," Sam explained. "He's not been formally charged with anything. If Niles will act as an informer for Interpol to further expose the activities of that damned London mob, they'll wipe his slate clean."

"I thought he owed the mob a lot of money?"

"I'm going to give him the dough to get them off his back on that," Sam said sourly.

"So it's up to me, is that it?" Morgan asked gruffly. "If I blow this thing wide open, Niles goes to jail and Nicole here goes back to issuing traffic citations, or whatever it was she did before she started toying with people's lives?"

"I should add one thing you might want to consider as you make your decision, Mr. Morgan," Inspector Danner said. "As of now we have no reason to disbelieve your story concerning your lack of involvement in the smuggling scheme, but should you choose to make the events of the past few days public, we would be forced to reconsider and bring charges against you as a participant."

"I can't believe you guys," Morgan said, outraged. "By what evidence would I be charged, might I ask?"

"You *did* announce to the world that you were Niles Kingman's partner," the Inspector reasoned. "It is circumstantial to be sure, but it could be very messy for you. You would not be allowed to leave France until the trial, some months from now, for instance. And there were some Italian pieces in the truck. The Italians might choose to extradite you for a trial of their own . . ."

"But first, of course, you would have to stand for your murderous assault on three officers of the law," Nicole said. Morgan stared at her in astonishment. To her credit as an undercover cop, she managed to keep her expression absolutely deadpan.

"Okay," he shrugged. "It looks like I have no choice. You win."

"That's just great!" Sam Kingman said jovially, slapping Morgan on the back. "And I want you to know that I intend to split the expenses for this whole Le Mans extravaganza right down the middle with you. We can issue some kind of statement about you and Niles reconsidering and deciding against the expansion plan—"

"What are you talking about, Sam?" Morgan asked cooly.

"Come on, kiddo," Kingman laughed uneasily. "You don't expect me to go through with this expansion thing now, do you? Not after all that's happened?"

"It looks like the conversation has moved into an area that does not concern me," Inspector Danner announced. "If you'll all excuse me, I shall return to my police work."

"Sam," Morgan began. "I made a deal in good faith with Kingman and Son, and I expect you to honor it." He winked at Nicole. "And I think Agent Houel will agree that it's vitally important to Niles' cover that everything proceed in a normal manner."

"Oh, but it is essential that Niles give the mob no reason to suspect anything is out of the ordinary," she nodded firmly. "Otherwise, it would do us more good if we prosecuted him and used him as an example . . ."

"For godsakes, Dad!" Niles blurted out. It was the first peep out of him since Morgan had arrived.

"This is blackmail!" Sam Kingman sputtered.

"Come on, Dad, just go along with Morgan!" Niles insisted. "You thought the expansion proposal was a good deal before all this happened . . ."

"I thought it was an okay deal . . ." Sam Kingman said. "You know, Morgan, maybe I could see my way clear to continuing this thing, if we could rearrange the terms . . ."

"Nicole, do you think they'd let Niles keep his cowboy boots in prison?" Morgan asked dryly. She had to bite her lower lip to keep from smiling.

"Dad—?" Niles didn't seem to think it was so funny.

"Okay, okay," Sam Kingman surrendered. "I'm going to play along, don't worry about it, Morgan. The deal we made will stand."

Morgan thought it over. What he was pulling on Sam Kingman really *was* a form of blackmail. "You can back out if you want, Sam," Morgan said quietly.

Kingman scrutinized him. "Don't kid a kidder, kiddo!" Sam abruptly laughed. "What about my son?"

"Niles will still get his second chance."

"I don't get it," Sam complained. "What's with you?"

"I've reconsidered, and I've decided that I only want to do business with somebody who wants to do business with me," Morgan said simply. "You once told me that you thought this deal was going to make you a lot of money. If you still think that way, fine. If not, walk away. No blackmail, clear enough?"

Sam Kingman nodded and was quiet for a few moments. Then he grinned shyly. "I guess all this trouble my son has gotten himself into flustered me. I wasn't thinking clearly. I *did* go over the paper on this deal. I originally thought that it was a potential gold mine, and now that I've come to my senses, I still do. He stuck out his hand, winking at Morgan. "You made a deal with Kingman and Son. Don't try to get out of it now. When we make a deal it sticks."

Morgan, grinning, shook hands. "If you're sure, Sam. . . ."

"Sure, I'm sure." He beamed at Morgan in admiration. "I've got a feeling I'm gonna be learning something about the car business this go-round. And I just hope Niles does as well. DonSport, America is gonna take off like a rocket."

"I think it will," Morgan said modestly.

"I *know* it will," Kingman firmly declared. "Niles

can be a jerk," he added, casting a withering stare at his son. "But one thing I got to say is that my boy's advertising and promotional instincts are right. That race tomorrow is going to be golden for us, absolutely golden—"

The race, Morgan thought. *Who was going to drive for him in the race?* "I've got to see Sonny."

"I'll call the doctor to tell him we're coming," Nicole said. "And then I'll drive you."

It began to rain lightly as Morgan and Nicole left the station by the back door and walked a block to where Nicole had parked her rented car. Morgan thought she seemed quiet, almost withdrawn, as she drove him the short distance to the doctor's small, but well-kept, two-story brick home, dwarfed by the other, far more stately residences on this wide, tree lined street.

"Well, I guess I'll see you tomorrow," Morgan said as Nicole pulled over to the curb to let him out. "That is, if you will still be acting as the press liaison for the race?"

"Oh, of course, I intend to," Nicole quickly assured him. "I hope you understand that as far as everyone is concerned, I must remain merely a free lance journalist. You can tell no one what has happened—"

"Except Sonny," Morgan said firmly.

"Except Sonny," Nicole reluctantly shrugged. She was staring out through the rain streaked windshield.

"Well then, I guess I *will* see you tomorrow," Morgan repeated.

"Morgan . . . I shall continue working with you, but I would like to continue . . . *other* things as well . . ."

She was silent for a moment. She seemed almost shy and embarrassed. Morgan realized that the forthright, sexually brazen Nicole he'd known was a fabrication; an alter ego, or whatever you wanted to call it, that was part of Nicole's cover. The woman Morgan was now seeing was the *real* Nicole Houel: shy, and somewhat unsure of herself, just like most everyone.

He kept his mouth shut, and listened to the rhythmic sweep of the wipers as he patiently waited for her to get her feelings straight and say what was on her mind.

"Morgan, my relationship with Niles Kingman. Well, that was in the line of duty, you might say. But *our* relationship . . . for me it was real." She glanced at him hopefully.

"I believe you," Morgan said gently.

"So, must it be over between us?" she asked sadly. She reached across the car's center console to take his hand.

"It's over already."

"Because of the way I acted last night? That was in the line of duty, Morgan," she pleaded.

He squeezed her hand. "I'm no longer angry with you about that, although I don't approve of the way you handled things. And I appreciate the way you tried to help me out with Sam Kingman, but—"

"It's Sonny, yes, darling?" Nicole softly asked.

Morgan nodded.

"Lucky girl." Nicole smiled ruefully. "Well, then, you should go to her, darling. She is waiting for you."

He was the lucky one, Morgan thought, getting out of the car, and hurrying up the doctor's flagstone walk. He was lucky *if* Sonny would still have him.

A very old and frail looking white haired woman answered the door at his first knock. She wore a black crocheted shawl over a gray wool dress that covered her from neck to ankles. She had a disconcerting, little girl's giggle as she greeted Morgan in French, stepping aside for him to enter, and introducing herself as Madame Tambay, the doctor's wife.

Morgan followed her through a small vestibule lined with mirrors and furnished with one of those elephant's leg umbrella stands, into the living room, which was all dark wood paneling, cluttered with bric-a-brac. Madame Tambay went off giggling, hopefully to fetch the doctor. Morgan, watching her go, got the feeling she'd thought this whole deal with Sonny to be the most exciting thing . . .

He spent a minute or so examining what had to be the world's most extensive collection of Hummel figurines, and then he was joined by a small, elderly, rather stout and prissy looking gentleman, a sort of senior citizen version of Hercule Poirot, who introduced himself as Doctor Tambay. He, too, spoke little English, but managed to make Morgan understand that the Mademoiselle entrusted to his care was in good health, but emotionally drained, and in a bit of shock concerning her experiences. He led Morgan upstairs, and along a poorly lit hall done up in green flocked velvet wallpaper, to what turned out to be a surprisingly cheerful bedroom. It had canary yellow walls, red area rugs on polished wood floors, vases of fresh flowers on French provincial furniture the hue and shape of tufted swirls of meringue, and a narrow brass bed. Best of all, the bed held Sonny, looking very small amid all the down pillows and bright, patchwork quilts pulled up to her neck. She was grinning at him and holding out her arms for a big hug, which Morgan was very glad to give her. Behind him he heard Doctor Tambay leave the room, quietly closing the door after him.

"I was so worried about you," Sonny sighed, holding him tightly as he sat down beside her on the bed.

"Worried about me?" Morgan laughed. "Who was the one who got herself kidnapped?"

"Yes, but they told me what was going on as soon as that shot they gave me wore off."

"That shot," Morgan growled. "How are you?"

"Okay. A little groggy," Sonny shrugged. "The Doc and his wife have both been just adorable to me. I feel like I've been having a cozy visit with the grandparents I never really had." She smiled, her eyes glinting. "Lots of tea with honey, and soft-boiled eggs and toast with orange marmalade . . ."

"Sounds great, all right." Morgan winced.

"How do you like my jammies?" Sonny asked, modeling her baggy, flannel long johns. The Doc lent them to me. They belonged to his son. You know, they have a flap in the back?"

"Steal 'em," Morgan said lewdly.

"If you're good, and tell me everything that's happened since I've been here taking the cure," Sonny insisted. Morgan told her what had taken place since the confrontation between Sonny and Nicole at his hotel room the night before. When he was done, she laughed. "I love it. I would have given anything to have heard Baldy say, 'I am zee police—' He really turned out to be a nice guy, you know. He came to visit me early this afternoon, in order to apologize for everything. He even brought flowers." She giggled. "You messed him up, huh?"

"Messed him up *bad*," Morgan chuckled. "You'll have to bring *him* flowers, now."

They both said, "I am zee police—" in unison, and laughed, and hugged.

"My hero," Sonny said softly, her breath tickling Morgan's ear.

"Sonny, about Nicole, and what happened the other night . . ."

"Shhh," Sonny shook her head. "It doesn't matter."

"When they told me you were kidnapped, and I thought your life was in danger, I realized how much you mean to me," Morgan said. He looked into her eyes.

Sonny sighed. "And don't you forget it," she said smugly. "Not that I intend to let you."

Morgan grinned. "After we're through here, we'll go back to Portofino for a few days, and you can remind me, a lot."

"About the race, tomorrow," Sonny began uneasily. "I'm sorry, honey, I really am, but I'm still just a little dizzy from that shot. I don't think that I had ought to drive . . ."

Now Morgan felt a little dizzy. "Of course you can't.

Don't worry about it," he heard himself say too heartily. What a phony.

"Morgan, you can do it," Sonny urged him. "This whole thing about not being able to drive competitively is in your mind. You can do it! You just have to *think you can!*"

Morgan looked doleful. "You used to work for the railroad?"

Sonny frowned. "Maybe I'd better drive, after all . . ."

"No way would I let you near a car in your condition!" Morgan said firmly. "I know I have to do it, and I will." He sighed. "I just have to deal with it, that's all."

"My hero," Sonny repeated, smiling.

Morgan winked at her. "I'll handle it." *Somehow,* he thought, cringing inside.

Sonny nodded. Then she yawned.

"I'll let you get some sleep," he said, standing up.

"I'll be there for you, tomorrow," she promised, settling back against the pillows and drawing up the covers. "To see you win." She blew him a kiss.

To see me something, Morgan thought. "Sleep well," he said and left the bedroom, closing the door behind him.

Sonny waited. She heard the taxi pull up and Morgan leave. A quarter hour later, she heard the stairs creaking as the doctor and his wife trudged up to bed. The house settled, then went quiet.

She hopped out of bed and danced barefoot around the room. *He loved her!* And not only did he love her, *he loved her enough to drive—*

That stuff about feeling weak and dizzy was a crock. The shot had worn off by the time the Interpol officials had come by, first thing in the morning, to explain what was going on. It had been easy enough to fool the good doctor into thinking she was still weak. He was a regular sweety-pie, but not the sharpest M.D. in the world. As far as he was concerned, it was perfectly normal for a female to be all traumatized and put into a tizzy by such a horrendous experience . . . Never mind the fact that she knew that she could have stuck it to those nerds in the Mercedes if they hadn't played dirty by shooting out her tires.

As easy as it had been to fool the doctor, she knew that it would really be a snap to play the convalescent with Morgan—

She also knew that the only way he was going to conquer his past was by being forced to confront his fear of competitive driving: sink or swim.

She knew he wouldn't sink. He was a hell of a lot stronger than he gave himself credit for being. Look at the way he rose up from that series of potentially devastating tragedies: the loss of his wife and the death of his mentor. Look at the way he had built a thriving business, and battled and conquered his alcoholism. Her beloved had proved every day of his life that he possessed the essential skills of endurance racing: bravery, discipline, and determination in the face of adversity. She knew what Morgan was made of; she just had to help him prove it to himself, just as she had known that the stubborn old mule loved her and would eventually come to that realization.

Her poor beloved was going to have a miserable night and an even more awful morning during those few hours before the race, Sonny thought as she got back into bed. But it was going to be for his own good. It really was. And she was sure that her father would have approved.

She thumped her pillows to get them comfortable and drifted off to sleep thinking that Morgan was obviously fated to have a member of the Thomas family—who dearly loved him—looking out for him for the rest of his life.

20

MORGAN GOT BACK to his hotel room around midnight. He immediately called Fabiano Manfredi to inform him of the loss of the Gatto. Fabi got a little hysterical until Morgan reminded him that it was *his* car, bought and paid for, not DeManto's. Fabi was still perturbed, but three hundred grand did a lot to soothe his nerves. He said that he'd have one of his works team come by to pick Morgan up for the race about an hour before it was to begin and hung up.

Morgan looked at his watch. The race would start at noon. He had eleven hours. He probably should try to get some sleep.

Sure. He began to pace the room.

How the fuck was he going to pull this off?

If he chickened out, the deal he had with Kingman might fold, and even more importantly, his relationship with Sonny would be tainted. Oh, she might not say anything, but Morgan could imagine the look in her eyes; he certainly didn't want to ever have to endure that look.

But if he raced, he was going to die. He knew that morbid fact as a certainty, knew it in his bones. He'd be in some tight dog fight for lead position with the other cars, and he'd make a mistake of judgment or technique and he'd go out in a cartwheeling ball of fire—

Like Lee—

He looked at himself in the mirror. His eyes were those of a cornered animal; he was pale, and sweaty.

He looked like a junky being forced to go cold turkey. In a way, he was. He was addicted to his fear, and tomorrow he would be forced to confront his addiction, with everything he cared about in the world at stake.

He had to beat his fear. He had to win that battle.

And then he smiled and told his mirror image, "But you don't have to win the race . . ."

It was absolutely true. He'd become so panicked that he'd forgotten the simple fact that this was merely an exhibition race. He had nothing personal at stake concerning where, or even *whether,* he placed at the finish.

What a fucking relief to have realized that.

He stripped down to take a shower before going to bed. It had been one hell of a day and with his relief had come sudden and total exhaustion.

He was going to stroke it tomorrow, he thought as he let the warm shower cascade over him, washing away his tension. He would hang well back in the pack—oh, maybe he'd make a few futile stabs at trying to take the lead—but they'd only be for show, to fool everyone watching . . . Except Fabi Manfredi. Well, fuck Fabi . . .

Except Sonny, the thought hit him. There was no way that Sonny would be fooled, and what she thought of him really mattered.

But he couldn't help that. She'd have to cut him some slack on this one. He would do the best he could, but as far as winning the damned thing went, well, there was just no way. He was going to stroke it; let someone who truly deserved it have the glory of the winner's circle. All Morgan wanted was to survive the day and get on with his life. Anything more than that would be a dream ending, and he's stopped believing in his dreams long ago.

He slept surprisingly soundly, and woke up at nine thirty, ravenous. He telephoned down to room service for a big breakfast and peeked out the window. It was a bright, sunny day. Grand day for a car race, Morgan thought jauntily. He pushed the thought from his mind.

Room service came while he was shaving. "Good luck, today," the waiter told him. Morgan grunted as he signed the check. When he was done eating he pulled on jeans, a sweater, and a leather jacket and checked the time. Quarter to eleven. Might as well go downstairs to wait for his ride.

To the circuit.

To the race.

He hurried into the bathroom, where he vomited. He looked at himself, gone pale and haggard in the medicine cabinet's mirror. He looked and felt like he was tripping. Talk about sixties nostalgia . . .

He brushed his teeth and went downstairs, dragging his feet like a man on his way to death row. Which he very well could be.

Fabi's man was waiting for him in the lobby, tapping his foot and looking impatient.

The drive to the pit garage located by the stands and the hour leading up until the race dragged on forever and flew by in an instant. Morgan felt as if he were trapped in an awful nightmare as he pulled on the flame resistant clothing emblazoned with DeManto insignias. He felt like telling Fabi that he didn't need the fireproof union suit, the stiff, dun-colored overalls, the socks, the gloves, the ski mask-like face covering, and the helmet. He didn't need all this stuff because this stuff was to protect the guys who risked their hides getting down and dirty out there, and he wasn't about to do that. This stuff was for a hot shoe driver. He was a stroker.

Settling into the red convertible Gatto (*"street-legal, just like you wanted, Donaldo, yes?"* Fabi had grinned), strapping himself into the contoured seat, running his gloved hands along the leather wrapped steering wheel, Morgan thought about the traditional procedure that was followed in the event of a crash somewhere on the 13.64 kilometer, eight and a half mile circuit: usually they first notified the family, and then the crew, and finally the spectators.

Morgan didn't have any family left to notify. There was Sonny, of course. She was out there somewhere, watching him. Expecting him to win. *Sorry, baby,* he thought. *You didn't pick a winner—*

Manfredi thumped the Gatto's roof, startling Morgan. "Donaldo, time to drive." His grin was huge beneath his handlebar moustache. "Good luck!"

Morgan brought the Gatto's engine to life, and eased the car out of the garage, across the slotted lines of the pit area, onto the track. He could hear nothing through his helmet beyond the Gatto's rumble, so the confused pandemonium that invariably preceded the start of every race silently unfurled through his windshield, like a movie without a soundtrack, or a dream: the stands were filled with spectators; helicopters hovered overhead to track and film the event; on the circuit roadway itself it looked like sale day at the shopping mall as the various automobiles maneuvered to find their assigned places in the starting grid.

The Gatto with its big, turbo-charged V-12, was assigned a spot at the front of the pack, wedged between a pine green BXI Leopard—talk about your fucking omens—and a German built, gleaming black Auden 1000, a particularly nasty looking bullet of a car with a full time, four wheel system of its own, and *twin* turbos. He knew the Auden 1000 well, and knew that it was just barely street legal, if you happened to live in Dodge City.

Morgan, engine idling, the sweat running down the back of his neck, watched the second hand on his watch as he gripped the wheel. Any moment now the race would begin: 25 laps; for the fastest cars, the race would last a little over two hours. He looked to his right and noticed the driver of the Auden 1000 staring at him. As Morgan watched, the guy flipped him the bird—

And then the Auden, and the BXI on his left, took

off like they'd been shot from guns. The race had started, and Morgan had let himself be suckered; the Auden's driver had deliberately distracted him so as to make him lose his starting position.

He slammed the Gatto into first and peeled out, over the hill and past the Dunlop Bridge. Due to his brief hesitation he was momentarily in the midst of the smaller-engined cars, but as he moved the Gatto through the gears the lesser vehicles faded, until Morgan was out ahead of them and in sole possession of an open stretch of road, ahead of everyone else but behind the Auden and the BXI which held first and second place, respectively. As they came up on the Tertre Rouge Bend, Morgan felt the impulse to floor the Gatto and put the fear of God into that Teutonic asshole in the Auden, but he reminded himself that right now he was in the safest spot of the dangerous, hurtling wolf pack of traffic that occurs at the start of any kind of race—be it auto or foot—until the participants stretch out along the circuit and begin the laborious process of going, or trying to go, the distance.

Anyway, what was the point of challenging the Auden in the first place? Let its driver play his games. Morgan was into accomplishing nothing but coming out of this race in one piece.

They hurtled down the Musanne Bend in exactly the same formation, with the Auden 1000 in first place, the BXI Leopard in second, and the DeManto Gatto in third. A cavalry charge of lesser Audens, BXIs, DeMantos, and other marques, brought up the rear. Morgan checked his speedometer—120 miles per hour.

They took the Indy Bend. Morgan realized that this Gatto's brakes had a tendency to grab, and that the car didn't stick to the road as well as the modified version he'd totaled last night: he'd have to keep that in mind.

At the Arange Bend, Morgan watched the BXI make a move to take over first position. The BXI tried to get past the Auden on the inside of the turn, but the Auden was clearly intent upon playing for keeps. Morgan watched as the black car closed the gate on the BXI by drifting toward the inside shoulder of the roadway. The Auden was suggesting that it was willing to suffer a sideswipe collision rather than allow the BXI to pass. The BXI was in no mood to call the bluff and fell back.

And then they were hurtling past the stands, which came and went in the blink of an eye, and soaring up over the crest of the hill, and down beneath the Dunlop Bridge: one lap down, twenty-four to go.

By Morgan's ninth lap he was almost starting to feel relaxed, in a tense, tentative kind of way. He'd been able to stay out of any sort of threatening situation by being satisfied to remain in third place, ahead of everyone else, but behind the Auden and the BXI, the two of which had exchanged first and second place several times. In all, the race had pretty much followed the pattern of the real 24-hour Le Mans by breaking up into a number of individual races between different classes of automobiles, all whipping around the same circuit.

It got a little dicey now and then when the various groupings of faster cars lapped the slower packs, playing a game of chicken with their fast brethren as they darted and weaved through the wolf packs of slower cars.

So far there had been no accidents, for which Morgan thanked God, and thanked Sonny, who'd had the smarts to remind him to make it very clear at yesterday's drivers' meeting that this was a publicity stunt, not a record book race; there was no point in risking lives. Everybody had evidently taken the advice to heart, except for the driver in the black Auden 1000. Several times he'd used his car as a weapon, threatening to physically plow into the BXI when it tried to pass. Usually the BXI backed down, but occasionally it succeeded in passing. On those infrequent occasions the Auden would suddenly accelerate to pass the BXI as if it were standing still. Morgan guessed the German driver was "sandbagging": reserving his car's speed, much as Morgan was doing with the Gatto. Of course, Morgan was sandbagging his car because he was a stroker, afraid of getting into a dogfight. The German driver was likely taking it easy, toying with the BXI in order to please the crowd. A good driver knows there's no point in sending the audience home early thinking that the outcome of a race is a foregone conclusion.

At the end of his twelfth lap Morgan pulled into the DeManto pit for his scheduled stop. He stayed in the car as the crew gassed up the Gatto and changed the smoking tires.

Fabi Manfredi was tight mouthed as he offered Morgan a cold drink.

"Seen Sonny?" Morgan asked as he sipped at orange juice through a straw.

"She's been around," Manfredi said brusquely.

"What's eating you?" Morgan asked, although he knew.

"The way you are driving!" Manfredi exploded. "Donaldo, what are you doing? The way you are stroking it brings dishonor on the *Professore* and the entire DeManto organization. It brings dishonor on yourself—" Manfredi was livid. "It brings dishonor on your woman! Sonny knows what you are doing—"

The chief mechanic yelled, "Go!" Morgan put the car in gear and peeled out of the pit without answering Fabi. He used the Gatto's reserve of power to slice through the traffic ahead of him, quickly making up the minutes lost in the pit. Before long he was back in third place, behind the Auden and the BXI, back to stroking it.

Morgan thought about what Fabi had said. He had no answers for the man beyond the fundamental truth that he simply did not have the balls to take the risks necessary to win.

At the start of the twenty-third lap the Auden's driver began to toy with Morgan. The black car purposely dropped back behind the BXI, to parallel Morgan in the Gatto. Morgan watched the driver give him the finger, shoot ahead to pass the BXI, then drop back to give Morgan the finger again.

The Auden's driver knew that he was stroking it, Morgan realized. The guy couldn't let well enough alone, Morgan thought, growing angry. The guy couldn't just be happy with winning the race; he had to humiliate Morgan over the matter. Humiliate him in front of everyone. In front of Sonny, who was likely disappointed enough in him.

Yeah . . . This German prick was starting to piss him off.

They were coming around past the stands for the start of the next to the last lap, when Morgan made his move, purely on instinct, without conscious thought—

Morgan blipped the Gatto's gas pedal, surging ahead of the BXI, and then past the Auden, whose driver had clearly been taken by surprise, to take over the lead, just as they passed the stands. Morgan had a momentary glimpse of what he thought was the crowd rising to its feet—

But then the stands were behind him, and he was under the Dunlop Bridge, and willing to chalk the image up to an overactive imagination, because the gleaming black Auden 1000 was coming up fast on his right, and Morgan knew that he was going to be in a dogfight, after all.

He knew one other thing too; underneath all that protective fireproof clothing, he had a raging hard-on. He glanced down at his crotch, grinning, thinking, *Welcome back.*

He and the Auden were neck-and-neck into the Mulsanne Straight, with the BXI a remote green splotch in Morgan's rearview mirror. At the beginning of the straight the Auden tried to pass on the left, Morgan swerved into his path to intercept, and the black car backed off. Morgan floored the Gatto, watched the speedometer's needle tickle 170 mph, and listening to the turbo howl, as he darted like a lightning bolt through the slower cars, lapping them yet again.

Fast mass, Morgan thought. That's what he was, and that was a vibrantly horny thing to be. He heard himself laughing, a trifle hysterically. He was in love with the Gatto, he realized. In love with its gift of speed.

He threw the car into a controlled skid to take the Indy Bend. The Auden stayed glued to his tail like Darth Vader on wheels, ready to drive right up his asshole if Morgan gave it the slightest opportunity. In the meantime, the canny driver of the Auden was letting the Gatto do the hard work of "drafting": breaking a path through the air, cutting the friction of wind resistance for him.

As Morgan passed the stands to begin the twenty-fifth and final lap he realized that it *hadn't* been his imagination; the crowd really *was* on its feet and cheering for both him and the Auden's driver; finally they were giving the fans the race they'd been promised. The one they'd come to see.

Then it happened, at the Dunlop Bridge, at the top of the curve that takes the stands straightaway over the hill. Morgan saw it only because he was just executing his "shut-off", backing off on the gas and blipping the brakes in order to make the turn as fast as he dared without risking a launch into space. Why the BXI driver chose that notoriously dangerous spot to make his move, Morgan would never know. Maybe the poor bastard also saw the crowd on its feet and hungered for their adulation. Morgan could understand that.

In any event, as Morgan slowed on his approach beneath the bridge, he saw a sudden flash of green in his rearview mirror. The BXI and the Auden were braiding across each other's 140-mile-per-hour-plus paths, struggling to take over second place, so as to be able to make a move for first place on the fast approaching, final, Mulsanne Straight of the race. The BXI tried a slingshot maneuver, drifting behind the Auden, and then moving out of the black car's slipstream and pouring on every bit of power to pass on the inside of that treacherous curve. This time, the Auden, perhaps sensing the desperation on the part of the BXI driver, did not try to shut the gate by veering towards the inside shoulder.

The Auden didn't have to.

The BXI swerved into the curve and Morgan watched, horrified, as the pine green car struck the inside guard rail, ricocheted across the track and then slammed into the outside retaining wall. Its image skittered out of sight in Morgan's rearview mirror as he slid into the Tertre Rouge Bend, and as the first tongues of orange flame began to lick at crumpled sheet metal painted that oh-so-familiar pine green.

Morgan had tears in his eyes. He felt like he was suffocating inside his mask and helmet. He took his foot off the gas, let the Auden pass him on the Mulsanne. *He couldn't make it,* he thought. *He just wasn't going to make it.*

And then, watching the Auden pull ahead, Morgan thought about what he'd managed to find the balls to do last night: he'd driven this same stretch of road—*in the dark*—lots faster than he was driving now, and then he'd purposely T-boned another car. He'd had the balls to outwit, outdrive, and then capture three trained, armed, police officers.

But he didn't do all that for himself; he did it for Sonny. Actually, he was in this fucking race in the *first place* for Sonny.

And for one other person, Morgan remembered. He'd dedicated this race to Lee Thomas.

Fast mass, boyo . . . Morgan could have sworn that he'd heard the Irishman's laugh echoing inside his helmet . . .

And then he was pressing down on the gas pedal, and overtaking the Auden as they entered into the Arnage Bend, and the homestretch. The Auden tried to bluff him, swerving into his path, preventing Morgan from passing on the inside. Morgan used his car like a boxer uses his fists, feinting an attempt to pass on the left, and then heel-and-toeing: working the gas pedal and brake with a single foot, to position the screaming Gatto on the Auden's right back bumper, and then *past* the sonofabitch, his twin turbos notwithstanding, because what Morgan did best was drive.

He never looked back, just pointed the Gatto like a gun toward the finish line, and didn't ease up on the gas pedal until he saw the checkered flag.

He slowed down, to shunt the Gatto onto the two and a half mile Bugatti circuit for a victory lap of sorts. The Auden, as second place winner followed him in, and Morgan let the black car draw parallel to him for a stretch. The Auden's driver waved, then touched his gloved fingers to his helmet in a bit of a salute.

Not a bad guy after all, Morgan thought.

As he swung back onto the Le Mans circuit, Morgan saw that some of the crowd had jumped the barrier, and Morgan had to slow the Gatto as he rolled into the winner's circle. As he shut off the engine Fabi Manfredi, with tears streaming down his blissful face, tore open the door.

The applause and cheers hit Morgan like a wave, almost knocking him senseless. Then the cacophony melded into a single forceful chant. At first Morgan thought he was hallucinating, but as he climbed out of the car and pulled off the helmet and the fire-mask, he realized that what he'd thought he heard was for real:

"DeManto/Morgan. DeManto/Morgan. DeManto/Morgan—"

"The driver of the BXI?" Morgan demanded.

"Walked away from the crash," Manfredi replied. "Poor guy blew a tire going into the curve."

Sonny, simultaneously laughing and crying, was suddenly in Morgan's arms. Fabi Manfredi, gibbering Italian as if he'd gone mad, was popping the corks on one after another bottle of Piper Heidsieck, baptizing everyone and everything in sight, including the car, with champagne.

"Bittersweet memories?" Sonny murmured teasingly to Morgan.

"Memories? Me?" Morgan said. "Didn't you know? I'm not into the past. I'm a today kind of guy."

Sonny hugged and kissed him. Morgan swept her up into his arms and spun her around. The cheering never stopped, as Manfredi blessed them with a champagne rain.